PRACTICAL CARE
OF THE
MENTALLY RETARDED
AND MENTALLY ILL

PRACTICAL CARE
OF THE
MENTALLY RETARDED
AND MENTALLY ILL

By

RUTHANNA PENNY, R.N., B.A.

Superintendent of Nursing Services
Porterville State Hospital
Porterville, California

With a Foreword by

James T. Shelton, M.D.

Superintendent and Medical Director
Porterville State Hospital
Porterville, California

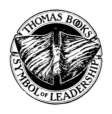

CHARLES C THOMAS • PUBLISHER
Springfield • Illinois • U.S.A.

Published and Distributed Throughout the World by

CHARLES C THOMAS • PUBLISHER

BANNERSTONE HOUSE

301-327 East Lawrence Avenue, Springfield, Illinois, U.S.A.

NATCHEZ PLANTATION HOUSE

735 North Atlantic Boulevard, Fort Lauderdale, Florida, U.S.A.

With THOMAS BOOKS *careful attention is given to all details of manufacturing and design. It is the Publisher's desire to present books that are satisfactory as to their physical qualities and artistic possibilities and appropriate for their particular use.* THOMAS BOOKS *will be true to those laws of quality that assure a good name and good will.*

Printed in the United States of America

U-6

To
The Nursing Personnel of Porterville State
Hospital whose devotion to the care of their
patients is a constant source of inspiration to me

FOREWORD

Man is upon the threshold of one of his most challenging areas of discovery—that of mental retardation and mental illness. Probably as much new knowledge has come in these psychiatric fields in the past ten years as in any other single specialty of medicine. With knowledge and the current "band-wagon" popularity comes danger. Some folks just haven't the experience or apperceptive basis to properly assess the complexities involved. Misconceptions, fears, and outright fabrications do much disservice to the thousands of knowledgeable and dedicated persons who have worked many years in these fields, particularly those who serve in our modern state mental hospitals.

There is little question in my mind but that the greatest treatment advances and most significant research and training of the professional is accomplished within the large state mental hospital. Here the highly trained physicians, psychologists, social workers, teachers and rehabilitation specialists work as a team to assist the most important person other than the patient, the psychiatric technician or nurse to do the job. It is to the nursing person that this book is dedicated; to provide practical methods to accomplish our primary goal—the development of each patient to his maximum ability.

Author and registered nurse Ruthanna Penny, with whom I have been professionally acquainted for over twelve years, is one of those rare nursing administrators who consistently demonstrates flexibility, adaptability and youthful vigor enabling the molding of a loyal dedicated nursing service of over 900 persons to serve the needs of 2500 retarded patients. She has drawn upon this extensive experience in composing this book. I note, with marked approval, that she begins with the retardate and in the initial chapter emphasizes that dictum which must always assume first priority in *any* hospital—the patient comes first!

Mrs. Penny opens by asking the age-old question, "What is

Normal?" Dr. Charles Berry, Medical Director of NASA's manned spacecraft center and personal physician for the U.S. astronauts reportedly said, "When we start to learn more about normalcy we will learn more about disease." In the field of retardation it may be paraphrased, when we observe growth and development in the "slow motion" of the retardate we will learn more about normal growth and development.

It is typical of Mrs. Penny to amalgamate the fields of mental retardation and mental illness in a common philosophy of care and treatment and yet deal with each in practical depth. We are appalled at the attempts of some misguided writers to dichotomize these two psychiatric fields of endeavor.

It is gratifying to note the emphasis placed on the importance of the sociopsychiatric history and the neurological examination in the diagnosis of mental handicap. The practical discussion of such problems as marriage for the retarded, unimportance of the "IQ" and consideration of "special problems" such as the blind, deaf, epileptic, and cerebral palsied, attests to Mrs. Penny's long practical experience with these concerns of our field.

Appropriately, nearly 100 pages are devoted to "caring for the patient." Step by step and hour by hour, suggested programming for habit training can easily be followed by the novitiate. Especially commendable are the detailed procedures given for feeding and prevention of deformities.

Those who work closely with hundreds of retardates are aware of such common problems as oral hygiene, clothing needs, pinworm and enteric disease, restraints and seclusions, "diversional activities" and industrial therapy. But no less attention is paid by the author to religious training, use of volunteers, proper record keeping (charting), and group and individual psychotherapy. Use of sociograms and case studies in visualization of a complicated process is so vital.

Besides the more conventional historical approach followed by the author in the section on mental illness, she gives us the story of the National Mental Health Association's bell symbol, "cast" from the chains and shackles once used to contain the "insane demons."

Emphasis of the high recovery rate of the mentally ill and comparison of operating costs between the "rich" general hospital per diem and the "poor" but surprisingly effective and efficient state mental hospital always bears repetition.

Description of mental health as more than freedom from disease is pertinent. Zest for life must be the core of mental health.

Mrs. Penny's use of clever illustrations for defense mechanisms and the major categories of the mentally ill adds a great deal of charm to this book.

There is much meat in the chapter on the practical discussion of treatment methods which emphasizes nursing procedures, therapeutic environment, group treatment, and motivational therapy.

The evolution of the psychiatric technician from the untrained caretaker, attendant, or aide, into a nursing person who is a mature, flexible, competent, therapeutically and patient oriented professional, is the message the author succeeds in putting across to the discerning reader. This book is a fitting successor to her first, *The Positive Approach.*

JAMES T. SHELTON, M.D.
Superintendent and Medical Director
Porterville State Hospital
Porterville, California

PREFACE

Gradual changes have been taking place in recent years in the composition of the population of state hospitals. This applies to those for the mentally ill and for the mentally retarded. An often quoted figure is that 50 per cent of hospital beds in the United States are occupied by the mentally ill patient. Figures that are not as well known are that for every 10,000 persons in the United States, 300 are mentally retarded. It is also true that greater public awareness and the development of community programs have decreased the likelihood for admission of the mildly retarded. The more active treatment and training programs in the state hospitals and schools have contributed to an earlier discharge of many of these patients; some, who in the past were expected to live out their lives in such facilities, today are soon returned to their communities.

On the other hand, younger and more severely retarded patients are admitted in larger numbers. Families often seek earlier admission for their children and public pressure is increasing to provide more beds for this group of the mentally retarded. A cross section of 100 of this group would show that about 10 per cent are mongoloid, about 30 per cent to 40 per cent have either epilepsy or cerebral palsy, or both. One half of the patients either cannot talk or are hard to understand. About 10 per cent have no useable hearing. Progressive medical programs and better legislative appropriations have contributed to the improved fortune and a longer life expectancy for these severely retarded children. The legions of individuals and organizations who are cooperating in upgrading the status of the mentally retarded citizens of the United States include organized parent groups, the medical treatment staff and nursing personnel of hospitals and residential facilities, volunteer and civic groups, sheltered workshop staff members, vocational training and counseling personnel, recreation and religious workers and legislators and administrators. Research workers, with the aid of research grants, are delving into the causes of mental retardation with the eventual goal of prevention of unhappiness in future generations.

The patient's relationship with the people with whom he is in daily contact during his hospitalization has been recognized as an important aspect of the treatment process. It is significant therefore, that the psychiatric technician perhaps more than any other member of the ward team, has the greatest exposure to the patient's day-to-day living experiences. His contribution in providing constructive relationships with the patients is basic to the treatment effort and it requires the most careful preparation and qualifications. The emphasis on this dimension of treatment, i.e., the psychiatric technician's training, has been stressed more in the last few years than ever before.

The material on group therapy will aid anyone faced with the challenge of doing *something* for the thousands of patients who remain in state facilities because even though the majority of authorities believe that many patients should not be in such institutions, the bare fact remains that there *are* thousands, who *will* live out their remaining life time in a residential facility of some type.

It is my belief as stated in my previous book, *A Positive Approach,* that the basic principles of patient care are applicable to all patients, be they mentally retarded or mentally ill, the variations in emphasis depending upon the individual.

An educational experience should be an enjoyable one, with a text that is easy to understand. This text has been prepared, therefore, with the hope that it will assist anyone faced with the task of caring for either those who are mentally retarded or mentally ill, and that it will in its own small way aid in eliminating the thought that any less fortunate individual be considered "hopeless."

CONTENTS

PRACTICAL CARE
OF THE
MENTALLY RETARDED
AND MENTALLY ILL

Chapter I

ORIENTATION

INTRODUCTION TO THE HOSPITAL

You have come to work for the first time in a hospital setting. You observe a lot of activity among many people: Doctors making their ward rounds, nursing personnel caring for bed patients, someone in street clothes directing some patients in a game, a man hurrying by with some plumbing equipment, a group of patients being shown how to care for a flower garden by a pleasant countenanced man, a truck driver unloading what appears to be food containers and yet another truck picking up bundles of linens from a building.

You hear a lot of conversation about team work, about interpersonal relationships and about different types of patients and you wonder just where you fit into this picture.

YOUR JOB

One of the first things you will be told, if not *the* first, will be that the patient is the most important person in the hospital.

The philosophy upon which any treatment program is based is that you must respect each patient as an individual, that no matter what the mental capabilities may be or how they are physically endowed, each and everyone is aware of kindness and understanding.

The mentally retarded patients are children mentally and in many instances have known no home other than an institution. To them you are a substitute parent, for many, the only "parent" they will ever know. In caring for and working with them you must be kind, patient, understanding and be able to call upon all the resourcefulness of which you are capable. You will be expected to use initiative and imagination in performing your share of the treatment program, as no two patients are exactly the same and the basic program may have to be modified (without taking unnecessary chances) to meet individual needs.

Many times the most important way you can help a patient is by just listening to him when he wants to talk to someone.

There may be times when a patient will call you names or strike out at you; an understanding of why he behaves as he does will help you to remain calm because, regardless of his behavior, no patient should ever be abused physically or psychologically. You must work to gain the confidence of your patients, as the success of any program will be dependent upon the faith and trust they have in you. Never betray their trust. Don't make promises to them that you cannot keep.

You, the psychiatric technicians, are the ones who are constantly with the patients. You must learn to observe and to report accurately anything pertaining to the behavior and welfare of the patients to the ward doctor. You must have a listening ear as well as an observing eye at all times because in a very real sense you are the liaison agent, or reporter in the "field," not only to the doctor but to an ever increasing number of therapists associated with the hospital.

YOUR ATTITUDE

You may hear the term "Attitude Therapy" or be told that you must have the right attitude about your work. What does attitude mean? It means how you feel about things and people; it is interwoven with your emotions, your behavior as it is reflected in your voice and posture and is a part of the treatment of every patient with whom you come in contact.

Everyone has certain emotional needs; indeed, there are four which are considered common to all of us: The need for love and belonging to a group; the need for self-respect; the need for respect from others and freedom to develop as an individual; the need for new experiences and a chance to succeed. Being aware of these will help you to have a better understanding of why patients behave as they do. By learning to understand, you will acquire the type of healthy attitudes a good psychiatric technician needs.

The way in which a patient is greeted upon admission to the hospital will often be the determining factor in how he will react to treatment. A friendly manner upon your part will help to dispel the fear and distrust which is felt by anyone faced with a new situation. The friendliness must be warm and accepting but must not lead to familiarity. You must not judge the patient's behavior. Remember that he behaves as he does because he is ill or does not know why he behaves as he does.

A loving attitude is one of the best therapeutic tools which you have in your possession. There is no patient, be it a retarded child or a psychotic adult, who will not respond to love. This does not mean that you should become emotionally entangled with the patients, but that you should offer them security, warmth and understanding. When working with the mentally retarded children, it will seem as though there is no end to their demand for love. They cannot be spoiled by too much love; but it is important as to how you show and offer it.

Your attitude will be judged by others by the way you adjust to varying situations, by the way you show respect for authority and by the way in which you abide by the rules and regulations which have already been accepted by the hospital community.

Your integrity and honesty will be reflected in how you handle hospital property and records. Information about the patients and their families will be available to you. Such information is always considered to be confidential and should never be divulged to the public.

You should keep your personal problems in the background. It is not the time to discuss your last date or the overdue payment on the old homestead when you are caring for mentally retarded or mentally ill patients.

The manner in which you wear your uniform and where you wear it are extremely important. The public is prone to judge the treatment program of a hospital by the way the employees appear and behave. Wear your uniform with pride and dignity.

The way in which you look upon the patient, the job and your own way of life may be summarized in the little poem *Take Time.**

*Squibb's Nurses Note: New York, November-December, 1961.

Take time to think
It is the source of power
Take time to play
It is the secret of perpetual youth.
Take time to read
It is the fountain of wisdom.
Take time to pray
It is the greatest power on earth.
Take time to love and be loved
It is a God-given privilege.
Take time to be friendly
It is the road to happiness.
Take time to laugh
It is the music of the soul.
Take time to give
It is too short a day to be selfish.
Take time to work
It is the price of success.

WHAT OTHER EMPLOYEES DO

There are many people other than the psychiatric technicians and patients in a hospital community; many in fact, working behind the scenes as far as personal contact with the patients is concerned. To understand what the other person does tend to produce more harmonious relationships, which in turn results in a truly therapeutic environment. A brief description of other employees' work follows:

The Ward Doctor

He directs and leads the treatment program for the patients assigned to his care. Both psychiatric technicians and nurses, as well as most patients look to him for loving care, counsel and guidance.

Social Service Workers

They provide the link between the patient while he is in the hospital and his family, the social and work resources of the community and the world outside. They are qualified by their training and experience to understand the emotional difficulties of children and adults, and the way that social and economic resources relate to the problems of individuals and families.

Psychologists

The clinical psychologist has four major functions: diagnosis, research, therapy and training. They aid in the diagnosing of a patient by giving a series of tests, such as an I.Q. test and in many cases aid in treating the patient by doing psychotherapy.

Hospital Dietitian and Staff

Food is an important therapy for the physical and emotional rehabilitation of the patient. All activities related to the preparation and service of food must be correlated and integrated by the chief dietitian with the total treatment program of a hospital.

School Teachers

Institutions for the mentally retarded have educational programs designed to meet the needs of the different levels of mental ability of the patients. The teachers usually have specialized training in their field.

Physical Therapists

This therapist is trained in the use of physical agents and in certain treatments of muscles and nerves. Through exercises and special means such as hydrotherapy (use of water) and light therapy, the physical therapist helps the patient strengthen muscles and nerves.

The Dentist

He is in charge of the treatment program caring for the patients' teeth, gums and related parts of the oral (mouth) cavity.

The Podiatrist

He is in charge of the treatment program which prescribes special care and treatments for patients' feet and the prescription fitting of shoes when needed.

Laboratory and X-ray Technicians

They carry out special procedures necessary for diagnosing and treating patients.

Rehabilitation Therapists

There are many types of therapies all of which have the goal of treating the patient through activity.

1. Occupational therapy (O.T.)
2. Recreational therapy (R.T.)
3. Music therapy (M.T.)
4. Bibliotherapy (reading)
5. Industrial therapy (I.T.)

Therapists with special training are usually in charge of each of the above.

6. Religious therapy
   Appropriate services are usually provided for the patients of the Protestant, Catholic and Jewish faiths.
7. Beauty and barber shop personnel.
8. Volunteer Services
   Volunteers offer assistance in many ways and although they never take the place of paid staff, they provide an all important contact with the community.

Laundry Staff

They are responsible for processing all soiled linens and clothing and getting them back to the wards for use in caring for the patients. They are indispensable to the hospital community.

Maintenance

Engineers, plumbers, electricians and many more keep the physical plant operating at all times.

Chapter II

NORMAL DEVELOPMENT

INTRODUCTION

Before learning about retarded children, it is only practical that you should first know something of what is considered a normal sequence of development of a child. We know that all children require training and guidance and that there is an average pattern in the progressive steps of learning to grasp objects, to walk, to talk and to behave in a socially acceptable manner. Knowing the sequence of development gives you a guide in knowing what to expect when you want to teach the child a new skill. Knowing what is normal for certain age periods will also protect you from disappointment, in that you will not expect the impossible of the child. These principles of

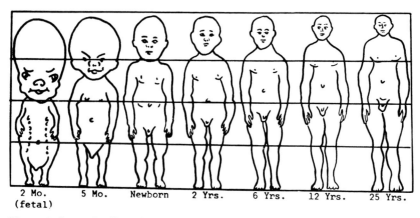

| 2 Mo. (fetal) | 5 Mo. | Newborn | 2 Yrs. | 6 Yrs. | 12 Yrs. | 25 Yrs. |

Figure 1. Stages In Growth: Relative proportions of head, trunk and extremities for different ages. (From Watson, E. H. and Lowery, George H.: *Growth and Development of Children,* 3rd ed. Chicago, Year Book Publishers, 1958.)

9

normal development can then be applied to planning a total care program for the retarded child.

A child's life begins when he is conceived, but it is not until the third month that the fetus definitely resembles a human being. Figure 1 shows the relative proportions of different parts of the body during fetal and postnatal life and indicates changes which take place with growth.

Each phase of development is influenced by the inter-play of inherited genes. The study of genetics, or hereditary, is a complicated subject and will not be expanded upon here; suffice it to say that a child inherits a large assortment of genes which determine his physical and mental make-up and a new combination of genes is formed with every child. That is the reason that no two children are exactly the same, even brothers and sisters.

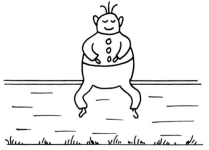

Figure 2. Heredity:

> Humpty Dumpty sat on a wall
> He was as wide as he was tall
> He didn't fret, nor did he gripe
> He knew this was his genotype.
> (or assortment of genes)

There are literally dozens of other factors which influence the mental and physical growth of the individual, some of which are: ancestors, cultural environment, family, illnesses of various types, endocrine gland disorders, sunshine, diet, education and exercise.

One could certainly say that the greatest gamble an individual ever takes is that in being born!

DEVELOPMENT OF MOTOR SKILLS

A summary of activities considered to be normal at various age levels are given below. Bear in mind that this represents the "average"

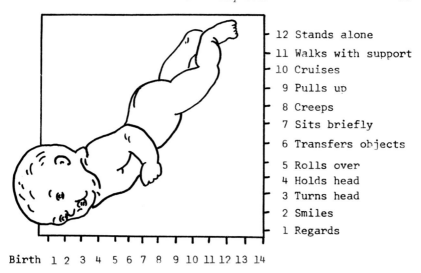

12 Stands alone
11 Walks with support
10 Cruises
9 Pulls up
8 Creeps
7 Sits briefly
6 Transfers objects
5 Rolls over
4 Holds head
3 Turns head
2 Smiles
1 Regards

Birth 1 2 3 4 5 6 7 8 9 10 11 12 13 14

AGE IN MONTHS

Figure 3. Developmental diagram for the first year of life. The infant's figure represents a diagonal line on which is plotted the progress of behavior (right of the diagram) against chronological age. (From Watson, E. H. and Lowery, George H.: *Growth and Development of Children,* 3rd ed. Chicago, Year Book Publisher, 1958.)

and that any individual could deviate from any one of the levels and still be within "normal" limits. Figure 3 illustrates the first year's progress.

4 weeks of age:
Hands tightly fisted. Head sags, tends to keep head turned to one side.

4 months of age:
Holds up head when sitting. Keeps fingers busy, wants to touch things.

7 months of age:
Can sit up in high chair. Bounces actively on standing. Bangs and shakes a rattle. Transfers a toy from one hand to another.

10 months of age:
Can sit steady. Creeps and pulls self to feet at rail. Will hold own bottle.

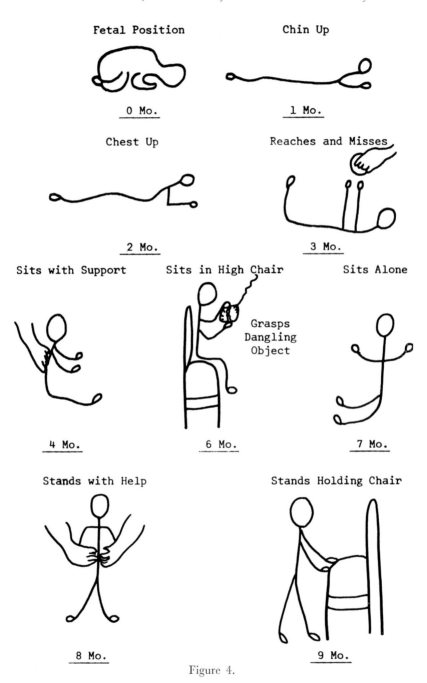

Figure 4.

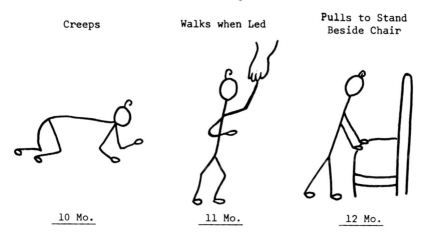

Creeps

Walks when Led

**Pulls to Stand
Beside Chair**

10 Mo.　　　　　11 Mo.　　　　　12 Mo.

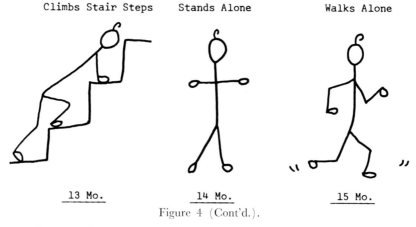

Climbs Stair Steps　**Stands Alone**　**Walks Alone**

13 Mo.　　　　　14 Mo.　　　　　15 Mo.

Figure 4 (Cont'd.).

1 year of age:
Walks with one hand held. Stands momentarily alone.

1 year 3 months of age:
Toddles about. Will creep up a stairs.

1 year 6 months of age:
Walks, seldom falls. Seats self in small chair and climbs into adult chair. Will hurl a ball.

2 years of age:
Runs well, no falling. Can go up and down stairs alone. Kicks a large ball.
3 years of age:
Alternates feet going upstairs. Jumps from bottom step. Can ride a tricycle, using pedals. Fine coordination is improving.

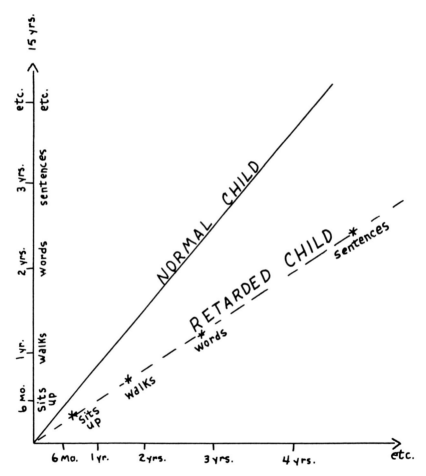

Figure 5. Chronological Age. A graph illustrating how the development of a retarded child can be compared with that of a normal child. (*Handbook of Psychiatric Management.* The Regents of the University of California, Berkeley, 1955.)

4 years of age:
Walks downstairs alternating feet. Hops on one foot. Throws ball overhand.

5 years of age:
Skips, alternating feet. Can stand on one foot more than 8 seconds.

6 years of age:
Advanced throwing. Ties shoe laces.

DEVELOPMENT OF TEETH

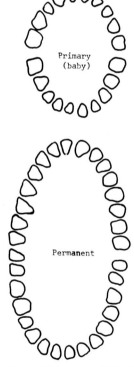

Primary
(baby)

Permanent

Figure 6. Time Table for Normal Eruption of Teeth:

Incisors	6- 9 months	1st bicuspid	9-11 years
Cuspid	16 months	2nd bicuspid	10-12 years
1st Molar	14 months	6th yr. Molar	1st permanent
2nd Molar	26 months	2nd Molar	12-14 years
Incisors	7- 9 years	3rd Molar	16-20 years
Cuspid (eyetooth)	11-13 years	(wisdom tooth)	

One of the most important steps in a child's development is the cutting of his teeth. If the first, or baby, teeth are not properly cared for, many problems may arise when it is time for the permanent teeth to come in. A child must have a good set of teeth with which to chew his food, otherwise he will not receive the full nutritional value from his food. Improperly masticated, or chewed, food can cause many types of digestive upsets such as colic in the infant or indigestion in older children.

A child may also have difficulty in learning to talk clearly if he does not have a healthy set of teeth. The development of a child's jaws is closely associated with how the teeth develop and grow.

A time table for the normal eruption of both "baby" and permanent teeth is given in Figure 6 (page 15).

DEVELOPMENT OF VOCABULARY AND SOCIAL ACTIVITIES

A child can communicate with you long before he can speak or use words; this is especially true with mentally retarded children. Adults working with any type of, or groups of children must learn their "language"! For example: a child may be in pain but is too young to tell of the pain, but he may be fretful, changing his position frequently and appear nervous. He may put a hand to the part, although if he is less than five years of age he will not locate the pain.

The sound, other than crying, made by a baby is the "Coo." The next step is the repetition of sounds such as "Ma-Ma." The progress from the "cooing" to talking so that he can be understood by those who do not understand his "language" is not completed until early childhood.

Even though a baby is capable of a wide range of sounds from the first month of life, he will tend to lose those which he does not hear in his daily life.

The increase in a child's vocabulary is often used as an index of his intelligence as well as of his physical and emotional development.

Some of the words and skills which are acquired by certain ages in a normal child are:

4 weeks of age:

Makes small throaty sounds. Stares indefinitely at his surroundings.

4 months of age:
Laughs aloud, smiles easily, coos, gurgles. An increased demand for sociability.

7 months of age:
Can vocalize m-m-m when crying. Takes foot to mouth. Reaches for and pats mirror image.

10 months of age:
Says "mama" and "dada." Waves "bye-bye" and pat-a-cakes. Feeds self a cracker and holds own bottle.

1 year of age:
Can say two words besides "mama" and "dada." Gives a toy on request or gesture. Takes a toy to the mirror. Cooperates in dressing. Prefers to drink milk from his cup.

1 year 3 months of age:
Knows four to five words including names. Pats pictures in a book. Points or vocalizes wants. Indicates when wet. Casts objects in play or refusal. Nursing bottle is cast aside.

1 year 6 months of age:
Has ten words. Looks at pictures and identifies one. Pulls toy on string. Carries and hugs doll. Toilet habits regulated in daytime.

2 years of age:
Uses pronouns, three word sentences. Verbalizes toilet needs. Pulls on a simple garment. Refers to self by name.

3 years of age:
Uses plurals. Gives action in a picture book. Feeds self. Puts on shoes and unbuttons buttons. Knows a few rhymes or songs. Understands taking turns.

4 years of age:
Washes and dries face and hands, brushes teeth. Laces shoes. Names one or more colors accurately.

5 years of age:
Knows four colors. Names penny, nickel, dime. Dresses and undresses without assistance. Asks meaning of words. Prints a few words.

6 years of age:
Uses a vocabulary of about 2500 words. Ties shoelaces.

Knows own right from left. Counts to 30. Differentiates, A.M. and P.M.

DEVELOPMENT OF PERSONALITY

Just as there are specific steps in acquiring motor skills, so there are stages in the development of an individual's personality. An individual's acceptance or rejection by society is generally determined by his behavior, which in turn is but an expression of his personality. It is a little easier to understand why a child, or an adult, behaves as he does if the basic processes of the development of personality are understood. (The following paragraphs are given only as a very brief summary; there are many excellent texts on child psychology for the student who wishes more information.)

Of the many schools of thought in psychiatry which pertain to the development of personality, one of those most frequently referred to is the psychoanalytic school which was originated by Sigmund Freud. According to his teachings the structure of personality consists of three basic parts: the id, the ego and the super-ego.

The id is that part of the personality with which we are born, is mainly biological in nature, is ruled by the pleasure principle and which says "I want."

The ego develops next as the result of frustrations and the facing of physical reality; it says "Better not because you will get hurt."

The super-ego is usually thought of as being equivalent to conscience, is cultural in origin and develops later than the id and ego. It says "You can't do that because it's wrong." There is conflict between any two of these at any time, this resulting in behavior. As only a small part of a person's mental activity is conscious, he is not always aware of what causes his conflicts.

The newborn infant is largely *id* and begins life completely dependent upon the adult who must satisfy its needs. The mouth is the baby's principal means of relating to the world; everything from fingers to toes, to food, to toys and clothing, eventually find their way to the baby's mouth. He "learns" through his mouth—not only the gratification derived from food but also the size, shape and texture of objects. This is called the *oral* stage of development and lasts about one year. The baby needs to be held when being fed, and loved and talked to if he is to develop normally. In most babies, there is a period when nothing seems to taste as good as the thumb. Thumb sucking was once severely frowned upon, but it is a perfectly normal type of behavior and is rarely, if ever, harmful to young babies. One of the most common causes for thumbsucking is thought to be an inadequate amount of feeding time at the breast or bottle. Other factors which might create a thumbsucking child are fatigue, minor discomfort or plain old boredom. Once you understand why a baby, or child, sucks his thumb, you can handle the situation according to its cause and stop having anxiety pangs about thumbsucking!

The exact age at which a child is conscious of his social environment is not known but he will smile in response to his smiling mother when he is about eight weeks old.

From one to three years the child is weaned, he cuts teeth and learns to show some aggressive behavior such as biting. Habit training in personal cleanliness begins during this period, the biggest task being that of learning control of his bowels and bladder. This training is seldom begun before twelve to fifteen months of age. This period of development is called the *anal* stage. The child soon recognizes the importance of correct disposal of his urine and feces. The ego becomes well developed during these years and the child, having learned how to either retain or rid himself of his excreta, develops a sense of power. Toilet training stimulates the development of the super-ego as the child realizes the social value of control of his alimentary tract. The stresses and strain of habit training are made more bearable for the child if the mother has made him feel loved and understood.

The years between three and six can be called the age of sexual awareness. As early as the last part of the first year the baby will discover his genitals the same way he discovered his fingers and toes; that is, by self-exploration. This is a normal occurrence. By the time the child reaches the potty-training age, he will explore himself with definite curiosity. Around the age of three the child begins to worry about why boys are not made like girls and vice versa. They may handle themselves a great deal, or masturbate, because they are preoccupied with thoughts about this difference in their anatomy. However, this is a normal step in development and should be considered to be relatively harmless. The only real harm which might occur would be from the emotional treatment with which an overly anxious adult might handle it. Even though the act of masturbation follows a definite course in many children and is a part of normal growing up, it is advisable to note at what time and under what circumstances the behavior occurs. If the adult's attitude is one of "Why?" rather than of "How can it be stopped?" he will be more relaxed about the "problem" of masturbation and will not feel the need to

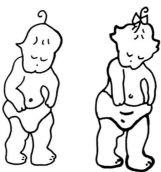

Figure 7. During the 2nd to 6th year the child becomes curious about his sexual organs and discovers the difference between boys and girls.

punish or restrain the child (which only tends to reinforce in the child's mind the ideas of something bad or wicked). Masturbation may be the sign of tenseness and anxiety at any age; preoccupation with it may be but one symptom of a larger emotional problem. Attempts should be made to change the child's environment through the provision of wholesome activities, suitable amusement, and arousing and developing in the child a healthy interest and concern about the welfare of others. These all would tend to divert excessive preoccupation with one's own body and welfare.

It is also during this period (three to six years) that the child learns the difference between male and female in regards to himself as related to the people who are important to him in his environment (father and mother).

The period of development between six to twelve years is a latent one in which curiosity about sexual matters is replaced by interests in learning, collecting, in adults other than his parents such as a school teacher, hero worship and joining a "gang," usually of the same sex.

Adolescence and the heterosexual stage of development occurs between the years of twelve to twenty-one. Adolescence is terminated when the individual is both sexually and socially mature.

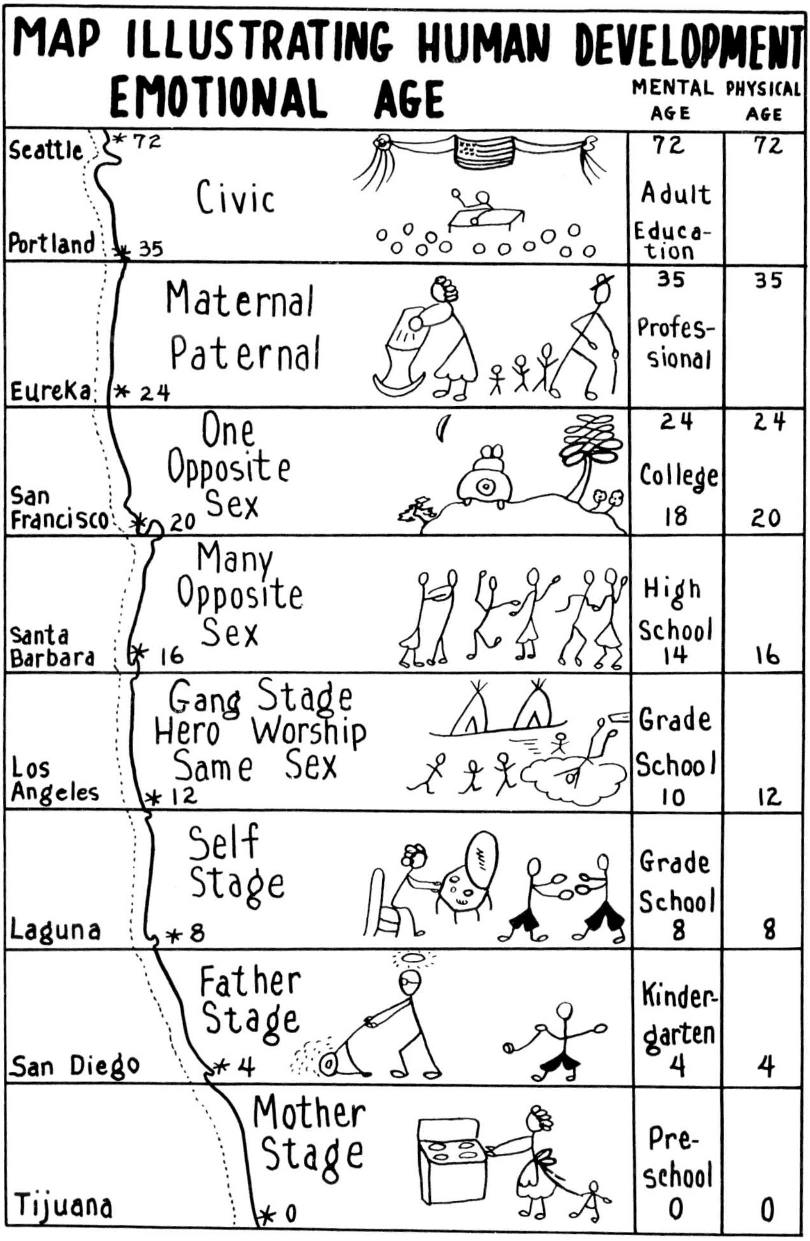

Figure 8. Map illustrating human development. From Madelene E. Ingram's *Principles and Techniques of Psychiatric Nursing*, 4th ed., 1948, Courtesy of the W. B. Saunders Company, Philadelphia, Pennsylvania.

Chapter III

MENTAL RETARDATION

F ALSE ideas about mental retardation include the beliefs a mentally defective child is:

1. Possessed by demons.
2. A hopeless case that should be put away and out of sight.
3. Cannot be trained.
4. Brings shame upon his family.

That it is a disease.

That it is based entirely upon a person's I.Q.

That it requires no special training or education to know how to care for mentally retarded individuals.

That there are no important areas of research in the field of mental retardation.

That mentally retarded persons possess strong criminal tendencies.

That the mentally retarded are over-sexed.

The only remedy is life-long segregation from society.

HISTORICAL BACKGROUND OF THE CARE OF THE MENTALLY RETARDED IN THE UNITED STATES

Mental defectives have been recognized from earliest times because of their inability to learn and to function in society as well as the majority of their fellows. In ancient times, they were commonly regarded as objects of ridicule and disgust and were often neglected, mistreated, or even eliminated, their treatment varying according to the dominant attitudes and superstitions of the society in which they lived. Later, when asylums were built to house the

22

insane, little distinction was made between the mentally deficient and the mentally ill and these two groups were frequently housed together.

The dawn of scientific and humane treatment of the mentally defective began about 1800 in France· It originated as a result of Dr. Jean Itard's interest in a "wild boy" who was found in the forest of Aveyron. Although Dr. Itard concluded, after spending five years methodically trying to educate this severely defective boy through intensive and extensive training, that his efforts were a failure he demonstrated that even idiots can be improved to some degree through training.

Itard's experiment not only demonstrated that psychological principles can be applied to problems of learning but marked the beginning of attempts to develop the limited potentialities of the feeble-minded to a maximum point of efficiency. His theory was: intelligence and thinking capacity could be developed by intensive sensory experiences and sensory training. Before his death, Dr. Itard handed down the account of his experiment to Dr. Edward Sequin, one of his pupils, who had become convinced of the improvability of mentally deficient children and who devoted the major part of his life to teaching and training such children. Sequin advocated what he called the "physiological method" which made use of very specific methods of sensory and muscle training as a basis for cultivation of the child's capacities to a point at which the teaching of speech, reading and writing might be possible. His philosophy of education was, with minor exceptions, quite like the principles advocated today for training mental defectives. He emphasized the education of the whole child, the individualization of instruction, the importance of rapport between the teacher and the pupil, the physical comfort of the child during the learning period, and the importance of beginning with the child's needs, wants, and desires before progressing to areas that are unknown.

Interest in the training of mental deficients soon spread through other countries, notably Italy, Switzerland, England, Belgium, and Germany. In Italy Montessori organized a school and a system of training based largely upon the principles formulated by Sequin. Decroly in Belgium, who believed that the best treatment of the mentally deficient lay in an educational program, can be considered one of the pioneers of modern methods of teaching mental defectives.

In the United States, interest in the care and treatment of the feebleminded developed soon after the beginning of the nineteenth century. In 1818 at Hartford, Connecticut, the American Asylum for the deaf and dumb admitted feebleminded children. In 1844 Dr. Samuel B. Woodward included in his annual report of the Worcester Hospital in Massachusetts a brief account of the training school for mental defectives in France. In 1845 Dr. Amariah Brigham, Superintendent of the New York State Lunatic Asylum at Utica, mentioned work done with the feebleminded in Europe and expressed a belief in the possibility of rehabilitating feebleminded persons.

Before 1846 no special provision had been made in America for institutional care of mental defectives. In that year, legislative action seeking public provision for mental defectives was initiated almost simultaneously in New York and Massachusetts. On May 8, 1848, the Massachusetts legislature voted an appropriation for the establishment of an experimental school which was opened in October of that year with Dr. Samuel G. Howe as director. This school, which was continued on a permanent basis first as the Massachusetts School for Idiotic and Feebleminded Youth and later as the Walter E. Fernald State School, may be said to mark the beginning of state hospitals in the United States although the first building in this country planned and built specifically for the feebleminded was started in New York in 1854. In 1848 Dr. Harvey B. Wilbur had opened the first private school for mental defectives in America at Barre, Massachusetts.

Pennsylvania was the next state to make special provision for mental defectives. A private school established in 1852 was incorporated the following year as the Pennsylvania Training School for Feebleminded Children. Soon after its incorporation, it was moved to Elwyn where it now is.

Other schools to open shortly were: The Ohio State Asylum for the Education of Idiotic and Imbecile Youth, opened in 1857; the Connecticut School for Imbeciles opened in the same year; and schools in Kentucky and Illinois opened in 1860 and 1865, respectively. Up to the year 1866 separate institutional provision for the mentally deficient existed in seven states of the Union, accommodating about 1000 patients in all.

The first institutions all began as experimental schools because of opposition on the part of the general public, the belief being that the feebleminded were beyond all hope of improvement and that efforts at training them were, therefore, futile. The organization and success of three of the first four American institutions was due largely to the personal influence and active aid of Dr. Sequin who had come from France to continue his work in this country on behalf of the feebleminded.

At the instigation of Dr. Sequin a group of outstanding pioneers in the care and treatment of the mentally deficient met in June, 1876, at Elwyn, Pennsylvania, and formed the association which has been in existence since that time and which since 1933 has been known as the American Association on Mental Deficiency.

The educational ideal which had been prevalent at the time of the founding of institutions in this country, an ideal unquestionably due to the influence of Itard and Sequin, gradually gave way to custodial care when it became apparent that the majority of institutionalized patients required such care. To meet the problems connected with the care of "low-grade" defectives, several special custodial asylums were established. The first custodial institution for low-grade defectives was founded in 1894 in Rome, New York, an institution which later became known as Rome State School.

A combination of several sets of circumstances led to what might be called an "alarmist" period in the care and treatment of mental defectives, particularly during the first two decades of the twentieth century. Binet's development of scales for the measurements of intelligence led to widespread testing and called attention to the relatively large number of retarded and deficient children in the population. Rediscovery of Mendel's laws of heredity, the rise of the eugenics movement following the work of the Darwin and Galton, and publication of genealogical studies of defective stock led to concern over the possible spread of mental defect through inheritance and was responsible for the advocation of segregation and sterilization.

The first attempt at segregation was undertaken in 1878 at the New York Asylum for Idiots where feebleminded women of child-bearing age were housed. Indiana was the first state to enact a human sterilization law (1907) providing for compulsory sterilization of "confirmed criminals, idiots, imbeciles, and rapists." By July 1, 1936, twenty-five states had eugenic sterilization laws on their books. While sterilization laws exist in twenty-eight states today, the laws are not operative in many because recent advances in knowledge have led to revision of the earlier attitude regarding the transmission of mental defect and the wisdom of sterilization.

At present, there is a noticeable trend away from custodial care back toward the educational or training ideal, for all grades of mental deficients, which was advocated first by Itard and Sequin. There is not complete agreement among educators as to the best methods to use in educating mental defectives but there is general agreement that the aim of education for mentally deficient children, whether in or out of institutions, is the same as that for any group of children. The aim is to teach the individual, insofar as he is able to learn, how to use all his capabilities and how to become a useful, socially acceptable member of his social group, whether that group be the community at large or the population within an institution.

There is also general agreement among educators of mental defectives that instruction should be adapted to the slow-learning ability of the child and that the program should be practical rather than academic. Emphasis has been given recently to the development of specific teaching and learning procedures for defectives with special disabilities such as brain injury.

The present-day program for mental defectives, having more of a psychiatric orientation than ever before in history, may be expected to meet the needs of defectives more successfully than they have been met in the past.

RECOGNITION OF MENTAL RETARDATION

Mental retardation should not be confused with mental illness. There is a vast difference between them.

A person who has been endowed with normal mental faculties may become mentally sick at anytime during his life due to numerous causes such as worry, shock and any one or combination of the varied pressures created by the tensions of present day living.

This may happen to a child as well as to an adult.

The mentally retarded individual is quite different. Their condition is the result of incomplete or arrested development of the brain. Mental retardation is not a disease in itself but is a symptom which may be seen in connection with many diseases. The process of making a diagnosis of mental retardation is a very technical one and should include:

1. A study of the background history of the child and his family.
2. A general medical examination.
3. Physical tests, which include measurements of the growing child.
4. Neurological examinations which test the responses of the nervous system (brain and spinal cord).
5. Speech, hearing and vision tests.
6. Psychological and psychiatric tests which include the I.Q., social maturity, emotional and personality factors.

Certain symptoms may be noted early in the child's life, such as convulsive disorders and physical handicaps in the new-born infant.

In the first six months of life, in severe cases of retardation, unusual placidity or extreme fretfulness are noted. The infant does not show an interest in his surroundings and he makes no attempt to sit up or to grasp with his hands. His head circumference may be below normal, or exceed normal size. These should be carefully checked by a specialist. It is unwise for a parent to try to make a diagnosis of his child's condition.

Social growth involves such things as the ability of the infant to occupy himself, to play while unattended, to demand personal attention, to follow simple directions, and to play with other children.

The child who is mentally retarded cannot learn as much as normal children. What he does learn comes slowly. By the time he reaches the age of four, there should be little remaining doubt about the seriousness of any physical or neurological condition. However, the retardation may not be clearly defined before the youngster is five or six years old. Sometimes parents do not realize that their child is retarded until after he has not been promoted through a grade or two at school. While it is recognized that many children are slow in school, they are not as slow in as many areas as are the retarded.

When the mentally retarded child grows up, he grows up in body only; mentally he will always be a "kid" but each one will have some unique quality that gives him a reason for his existence.

THE ADOLESCENT WITH MENTAL RETARDATION

"Psychologically, the adolescent has to learn to know himself and what he is striving to express. The adolescent with mental retardation because of his delayed development has evolved little identity; he often doesn't know where or how he fits into the world around him, and his family doesn't either.

"Usually his vocabulary is limited, making it doubly difficult for him to share his feelings, ideas, hopes, sorrows, and fears with anyone else. Those around him tend to think of him in terms of what he cannot do; he is thought of as a retardate rather than as a person who has retardation. He often realizes that he has been stereotyped as someone to be afraid of; on the playground at school he may hear younger children express their fears of him.

"Physical growth has changed him into an adolescent, but because of his slow mental development, the emotional development of childhood is not completed.

"As with all adolescents, the behavior of the adolescent with retardation is determined by what has evolved in his total life. For example, some parents overly indulge their adolescent with retardation in the attempt to protect him from harm. Like a 'sick child,' the child with retardation tends to get more attention than his siblings; parents often make unnecessary allowances for his condition. This causes the adolescent to develop a sense of isolation and feeling of difference from others. A sixteen-year-old boy with Down's Syndrome told the nurse he couldn't go to see the counselor because he was 'special.' She asked what he meant and he replied 'when you are special, you can't do what the others do.'

"Some parents are concerned because their child greets people by embracing them or attempting to sit in their laps. When the child is over-protected and kept from social contacts, his childish behavior is likely to persist. Parents often try to 'keep the child busy,' setting perfectionist standards of prescribed tasks. Too often these adolescents are routinely expected to set the table, wash the dishes, empty the trash, and so on, without the opportunity to 'take turn' and be included in the family. A different kind of problem is created by those parents who fear that the child will not be able to accomplish even simple tasks. The result of too much perfectionism or a demanding attitude on the part of the parent can create many problems for the adolescent with retardation. For example, normal adolescents do not cheerfully assume the tasks of washing dishes and setting the table; in the same manner, the adolescent with retardation often resists these tasks. Even the very limited of these young people need at least the choice of sometimes deciding what they will do next, freedom about doing tasks that are not immediately imperative, and approval for tasks well done.

"The nurse can help parents understand that an adolescent with retardation can often learn to do his own laundry, cook, clean, travel on public transportation, and earn money in sheltered situations. His skills can become a source of pride to him and his family. Although the nurse may recognize abnormal fears in some parents, she should focus her attention on tasks which give both the parents and the adolescent success.

"Adolescents with retardation need socialization and recreation as well as work. Parents need the support of the community in establishing recreation programs in public parks, swimming lessons at the Y and workshops for the adolescents. The nurse needs to be familiar with community, state and federal resources so she can help the family face realistic alternatives for the future. If she feels that the parents would accept skilled counselling, she may be able to make referral for help. Parents are naturally reluctant to face the limited future. But these young adolescents with retardation need honest answers when they ask 'When can I drive the car?' or 'Can I marry?' With a foundation of respect for what they can do, and help in recognizing that not everyone they know can drive or has married, they appear to accept these limitations.

"Parents need all the encouragement they can get to keep from further retarding their children by unrealistic protection."*

---

*Hillsman, Gladys M., R.N., Nursing Consultant, Division of Material and

MARRIAGE FOR THE MENTALLY RETARDED

This is a question which is frequently asked: Can, or should, mentally retarded individuals be permitted to marry? As a Psychiatric Technician, or any other personnel, caring for the mentally retarded, you may be called upon for an answer from your patients or from your fellow citizens in the community.

Marriage is usually considered to be a civil contract, and as such is forbidden for the retarded person in three states, and depending upon how the state laws are interpreted, is also forbidden in over a dozen other states. The main reason for a law preventing marriage among the retarded is allegedly to prevent the birth of children to parents who cannot care for them, or to prevent the hereditary types of mental retardation from being reproduced.

Just as there has been a growing recognition of the ability of the mentally retarded to assume an economic role in the community, there is an increasing recognition that some of them can also provide for a family if they are permitted to live a normal life. Every candidate for marriage would require careful individual evaluation before being permitted to take such a momentous step. Factors that should be considered, other than the I.Q., would be the individual's emotional stability, dependability, physical status and his judgmental abilities, even though in some states "the courts take the view that to consent to marriage does not require as great a mental capacity as that required to handle business affairs."

For the mildly retarded and borderline retardate, there have been studies in recent years that reveal them as being capable of having a satisfactory married life.

The retarded person is as capable of emotional feelings and responses as you are and should be legally entitled to the benefits of marriage. A married couple, even when both members are mentally retarded, may be quite capable of having a family, if there are not too many children. On the other hand, many authorities

---

Child Health, Ohio Department of Health, Columbus, Ohio.

Ross Laboratories, Columbus, Ohio, publishers of Pediatric *Nursing Currents,* September, 1964.

are of the opinion that while marriage provides for normal sexual gratification, the mentally retarded should not have children.

The prevention of parenthood implies sterilization and compulsory sterilization has long been frowned upon by many groups. However, Medora Steedman Bass has stated:

"Sterilization protects society and furthers public policy by providing defectives with an opportunity for normal rather than deviant sexual gratification, by tending to discourage illegitimacy and by preventing the birth of possibly defective legitimate children. The objection to sterilization by one religious group are well known, but it is less well known that the National Council of Churches, the Episcopalian, Methodist and Lutheran Churches, and some Jewish congregations have approved of voluntary sterilization under certain conditions. Since sterilization would be on a voluntary basis, no one could be forced to have the operation if it was inconsistent with his religious beliefs.

"An attempt to liberalize the law was made recently in Pennsylvania by a group of individuals interested in the welfare of the retarded. They called for exemption from the marriage prevention laws any retardates who had been sterilized. The action of this group could serve as a model for those in other states who may want to liberalize the laws so that the mentally retarded may enjoy the stabilizing influence of the marriage relationship."*

THE I.Q.—WHAT DOES IT MEAN?

Introduction

You get the I.Q. (intelligence quotient) of a person by doing simple arithmetic: Divide your mental age, or M.A. (functional level as determined by an intellectual maturity test), by your chronological age, or C.A. (how old you are) and multiply by 100.

What happens after you get it is anything but simple, perhaps even quite frightening, for many people. Our society places a high premium on intelligence and has, historically, used the technique of "out of sight, out of mind" in caring for the mentally retarded.

The intelligence quotient of a patient is no longer looked upon

---

*Reprinted by permission from *Mental Retardation*, 1964 (August) 2, 4, 198-202, a publication of the American Association on Mental Deficiency.

as a measure of limits; indeed, to tie a child to a number is dangerous. Just to say that a child has an I.Q. of 70 or of 130 doesn't really mean much. Of much greater significance would be the measurement of his "social quotient," that is, how does he adapt to the regulations imposed by society, such as bladder and bowl functions or his eating habits.

You may then ask, of what value then, is the measuring of a child's intelligence? It gives the parent, as well as the school teacher, an idea of what can be expected of the child. And it provides a guide as to the child's potential ability for the physician, the social worker, the psychologist or anyone whose task it may be to interpret to a parent what the future may hold for his child.

HISTORICAL BACKGROUND OF THE MEANING OF I.Q.

It was assumed that all that was required to establish a diagnosis of "Mental Deficiency" was the giving of an appropriate I.Q. test. Closely associated with this concept was the idea that a given individual's I.Q. is fixed and constant throughout his entire life.

In British literature the term "mental deficiency" is usually used as a substitute for feeblemindedness in the generic sense, the word "feeble-minded" being applied by British workers to what American workers call the moron.

In 1934 the American Association on Mental Deficiency adopted a modification of the psychological criteria for grading mental defect in which the mental age of an individual was equated with a given I.Q. average. An I.Q. of less than 20 equals a mental age of less than three years, an I.Q. from 20-49 equals a mental age of three to seven years and an I.Q. of 50 or more equals a mental age of eight years or upwards. They also state: "As a rule the upper limit for a diagnosis of mental deficiency should be an I.Q. of 69, but this limit should not be adhered to in cases where medical, social and other factors clearly indicate that the patient is mentally defective."*

The American Psychiatric Association classifies the degree of retardation as mild, moderate or severe.

---

*Deutsch, A.: *The Mentally Ill in America,* 2nd ed., New York, Columbia University Press, 1952, p. 363.

Changing Terminology

"*Intelligence* is often confused with the level of education which a child is able to achieve. It would be nearer the truth if it was said that the higher one goes in school, the higher the I.Q.'s to be found. This in part is due to the fact that those with lesser potentialities, without the opportunity and without the goals and aspirations drop out of school sooner."*

Traditionally, psychologists and educators have grouped the mentally deficient in three or four categories. In reality there is little or no real difference between a child at the top of one grouping and the child at the bottom of the next highest group.

Idiot   I.Q. 0-25—severely retarded.

Imbecile   I.Q. about 25-50—moderately retarded.

Moron   I.Q. about 50-69—mildly retarded.

Borderline I.Q. from about 70 to about 80. This group has a final mental age of about $10\frac{1}{2}$ years to 12 years. Many in this group will need special attention in public schools but as adults will be self-sufficient in terms of making a living.

The *social criteria* is perhaps the most important of all because if the mentally retarded individual cannot be trained to conform to the needs of his society, he must spend his life in a hospital or other facility.

The *mildly retarded* individuals usually manage to maintain themselves in school and eventually in society without too much specialized attention. They are the slow learners in school but "special classes" within the regular grades are considered in many communities as adequate educational coverage.

The *moderately and severely retarded* groups present the major social problem. They are referred to as the mentally handicapped, mentally deficient, the feebleminded or the mentally retarded. The term *mentally retarded* has been most widely used in recent years because of its acceptance by parent groups.

A listing of recent changes in terms give the following:

Moron   —becomes "educable" group.

Imbecile—becomes the "trainable" group.

Idiot   —becomes the "total care" group.

*Heiser, Karl F.: *Our Backward Children*, New York, Norton and Co., 1953.

The most recent changes in terminology pertaining to measured intelligence and diagnostic classifications have been prepared and issued by the *American Association on Mental Deficiency* in 1959. The term *adaptive behavior* refers primarily to the effectiveness with which the individual copes with the natural and social demands of his environment. "Since these standards vary with age, adaptive behavior is always evaluated in terms of the degree to which the individual meets the standards of personal independence and social responsibility expected of *his* chronological age group.

TABLE I

Pre-School Age 0 - 5 Maturation and Development	School-Age 6 - 21 Training and Education	Adult 21 Social and Vocational Adequacy
Level I		
Can develop social and communication skills; minimal retardation in sensori-motor areas; rarely distinguished from normal until later age.	Can learn academic skills to approximately 6th grade level by late teens. Cannot learn general high school subjects. Needs special education particularly at secondary school age levels. ("Educable")	Capable of social and vocational adequacy with proper education and training. Frequently needs supervision and guidance under serious social or economic stress.
Level II		
Can talk or learn to communicate; poor social awareness; fair motor development; may profit from self-help; can be managed with moderate supervision.	Can learn functional academic skills to approximately 4th grade level by late teens if given special education. ("Educable")	Capable of self-maintenance in unskilled or semi-skilled occupations needs supervision and guidance when under mild social or economic stress.
Level III		
Poor motor development; speech is minimal; generally unable to profit from training in self-help; little or no communication skills.	Can talk or learn to communicate; can be trained in elemental health habits; cannot learn functional academic skills; profits from systematic habit training. ("Trainable")	Can contribute partially to self-support under complete supervision; can develop self-protection skills to a minimal useful level in controlled environment.
Level IV		
Gross retardation, minimal capacity for functioning in sensori-motor areas; needs nursing care.	Some motor development present; cannot profit from training in self-help; needs total care.	Some motor and speech development; totally incapable of self-maintenance; needs complete care and supervision.

Intelligence as measured by the figures of an I.Q. test will correlate with these levels."*

Special Education

"This field of specialization has been in existence for over 50 years, but legislation passed that long ago has not as yet successfully included all the children for which it was meant. By 1950 no State had laws specifically encouraging local districts to provide for the 'trainable' mentally retarded child,"† although there has been a new trend during the past ten years to make provisions for this group of children. A specific example is the State of California, whose State Legislature has set forth in its Welfare and Institutions Code provision, as it pertains to the hospitals for the mentally retarded, for the "care, training and education of the persons committed thereto."

WHAT CAUSES MENTAL RETARDATION?

Mental retardation can strike any family; it is quite impartial in its selection. Doctors do not always know why, how or when it will happen.

Mental retardation originates during the developmental period and is associated with impairment in one or more of the following: maturation, learning and social adjustment. Synonymous terms for mental retardation include mental deficiency, backward, slow learner, exceptional, and the least desirable term "feeble-minded."

Although mental retardation is not a disease in itself, there are sixty to seventy diseases and/or body disorders which can each play a great part in causing it. The retardation is a symptom of an underlying brain disorder. The incidence of mental retardation is estimated between 1 per cent to as high as 25 per cent but the generally accepted incidence is that 3 per cent of the country's population has some degree of mental retardation. Less than 1 per cent of the population is believed sufficiently retarded to require twenty-four-

---

*Sloan, William, Editor: Manual on terminology and classification in mental retardation. Amer. J. Ment. Defic., 64; 63, 1959.

†Rosenzweig, L. E., and Long, Julia: *Understanding and Teaching the Dependent Retarded Child*, Darien, Conn., Educational Publishing Corp., 1960, p. 12-13.

hour hospital care. The vast majority of retarded people in the United States look no different than you or I. However, there is a small group, about 12 per cent to 15 per cent of the entire number of mentally retarded, which has definite physical traits.

It is not the intent of this text to teach patient care by diagnostic label. Your ability to give tender loving care to a patient would not vary if you knew that his retardation was due to "Encephalopathy Associated with Pre-Natal Infection"! However, standard classifications can be used as guides and as an aid in communications. Psychiatric Technicians and other members of the treatment team caring for the mentally retarded should have an awareness of a few of the more commonly used "labels." In this way they can share in and benefit from discussions concerning patients and their treatment.

A short list of diagnostic, descriptive terms and a brief explanation of each is given in Appendix E.

PATIENTS WHO HAVE SPECIAL PROBLEMS

Introduction

There are many mentally retarded patients who have additional handicaps, such as being blind, being unable to hear, and being subject to having seizures, or are physically crippled due to cerebral palsy. Some are so unfortunate as to have a combination of these conditions. The psychiatric technician must endeavor to learn as much as he can about each individual patient and how best to give nursing care to meet the needs of each patient. The ward doctor, the registered nurse and many special therapists are usually available for assisting and teaching the psychiatric technician how to best cope with the varied problems.

Deaf Patients

The deafness may be complete or only partial. The technician should learn the tone of voice to which the patient with partial hearing will respond, then use that tone. Otherwise, you may find yourself shouting or speaking in an unnecessarily loud voice. Some deaf patients can learn to read lips. When talking to these patients, you must face them, speak slowly but normally, without uncalled for facial expressions. Some patients, unable to express themselves verbally, will use a modified type of sign language to make known their needs.

Sometimes the technicians who are in close contact with the patients all the time will note some action or behavior on the part of a retarded deaf patient which leads him to believe that the patient could perform at a higher level if he had a hearing aid. Perhaps the patient may never have had an audiometric test, or the testing of the degree of hearing by an audiometer (this is done by a specially trained person). The psychiatric technician could call the patient to the ward doctor's attention who might in turn re-examine the patient and order the special test.

Blind Patients

In my opinion, the handicap of blindness is more tragic than that of deafness. It is impossible for a person who is blind from birth to imagine the world of the sighted. For those who lose their sight in later years, there is some degree of memory for what has been seen. Only teachers with special training and experience in working with blind children can be familiar with their lack of mental contacts in certain areas to be able to teach them properly.

The psychiatric technician can do much for the blind patients on his ward. The blind child needs to be talked to even more than those who can see. He needs to be given experiences through sound as well as through the sense of feeling. Providing as much of these as you can will aid in preventing the dull, passive expression and posture which is often seen on the blind person. Many blind patients can learn to do a great deal for themselves if trained to follow an established routine.

Ideally, blind patients, if ambulatory, should be in a ward environment in which the furniture is not moved about. The patients can then learn the location of all objects and be able to avoid bumping into them, or tripping over them and falling. Toys and other small objects should not be left lying about on the floor for blind, or other, patients to trip over and fall. Usually the blind patients are not segregated on a ward to themselves, but are placed on wards with patients who are sighted. This of course means that furniture, and everything that is movable, usually gets moved about. Fellow patients many times can be quite helpful in assisting the psychiatric technician with the care of the blind patients. As with all retarded patients, the more that the technician can train the blind patient to do for himself, the lighter will be his work load.

Patients Who Have Spastic Paralysis

Cerebral Palsy patients are frequently called "spastics" or described as having "spastic paralysis." What causes cerebral palsy is not definitely known, but it might be caused by an injury to the brain at birth or by an infection which affects the brain later in the child's life. The condition results in disturbances in the action of the various muscles of the body and there is some degree of mental retardation in about 75% of cerebral palsied individuals. The actual symptoms will depend upon the area in the brain which has been damaged. Three types are generally described: the spastic, the athetoid and the ataxic.

The Spastic

1. These patients have a stiff gait with the toes seeming to catch together and drag, or they may walk on their toes. Their legs may want to cross when they try to walk.
2. The finger muscles, as well as the muscles of any affected part, are tight and rigid at all times. Without adequate treatment the patient may become bedfast, or at best, confined to a wheelchair.
3. The tendency to have seizures is more common in this type.
4. Many are cross-eyed.
5. These patients have great difficulty in talking, the words being spoken slowly and with problems in the pronunciation.
6. The patient is usually very apprehensive, or fearful, because he associates contraction of his muscles with being hurt.
   a. Loud noises, loss of support, meeting strangers, or any unusual or new situation, may cause fear which in turn stimulates the muscles, causing them to contract violently.
   b. Because of this fear these children seem to avoid any attention which would lead to being touched or anything new or different. But you cannot avoid them.

The Athetoid

1. These patients have an almost continuous, slow, purposeless movement of the muscles of the toes or fingers, or of the limb or of almost the entire body. They have a degree of the stiffness of the "spastic" plus the motion.
2. Many have a severe hearing loss or are totally deaf.
3. Lacks confidence since he is always in motion and cannot be sure that he will accomplish a desired act. Whenever he falls he doesn't hurt himself since he doesn't become rigid, so he does not develop fear like the spastic.
   a. Is often outgoing and friendly, has a cheerful disposition and will enter into activities with others.

The Ataxic

1. These patients have a disturbance in their sense of balance and walk with a staggering gait.
2. May have nystagmus, or a continual movement of the eyeballs.
3. The different types also have different emotional needs. Differences concerning the need for love are:
   The spastic and the ataxic children do not as a rule like demonstrations of affection.
   Fondling and embracing sets off a "stretch reflex" causing vigorous muscle spasm.
   a. This makes the experience unpleasant and it becomes associated with dissatisfaction.
   b. The spastic child wants only love that gives him a feeling of security and protection.
   For the ataxic child anything which involves a shift in position such as rocking or tossing, or any motion which disturbs his equilibrium, or sense of balance, increases his dizziness to a painful degree.

The athetoid patients are usually very affectionate, want attention and like to be fondled and caressed.

The ideal situation for the care and training of these patients would be a unit or ward apart from the noise, the activities and the demands of the physically normal patient population of an institution.

Just what the "spastic" patients will be able to accomplish will depend upon their mental ability, the degree of physical defect and their age when treatment begins. Better results will be achieved if the patient can understand what he is told to do. Basic principles of treatment are relaxation and muscle training. In most hospitals emphasis is placed on physical therapy to establish the muscle training, relaxation and formal exercises. Every patient should be trained to make use of whatever potential he has, and inasmuch as most institutions do not have many physical therapists or occupational therapists, the psychiatric technician must do what he can, in addition to the regular nursing care. The technician should call upon the physical therapist and/or occupational therapist for assistance and instruction as to how to carry on with caring for the special problems pertaining to the "spastics." One of the problems is the modifying of spoons and other utensils used in eating. Spoon handles can be modified in several ways.

PATIENTS WHO HAVE SEIZURES

There are many reasons why a patient may have a seizure, or convulsion. The seizure is usually a symptom of the underlying cause producing the illness. Epilepsy causes a large percentage of the seizures which occur among mentally retarded patients. The kind of seizure the patient has will depend upon the type of epilepsy which he may have.

Idiopathic Epilepsy

The cause is unknown but the pattern of the convulsion is always characteristic. The patient may have a grand mal (big) or a petit mal (little) seizure. Sometimes the patient has a warning sensation, such as a "funny feeling in the head" and can tell you, but it is the exception if a mentally retarded patient can verbalize this to you. Sometimes the patient will just make a sound like "aaah." To be able to protect the patient from injuring himself, the psychiatric technician must be able to recognize the signs of an impending seizure.

Grand Mal

1. The aura, or the warning.
2. Fall, which may occur anywhere.
3. Tonic phase, or when the patient becomes completely rigid for two or three minutes, or less.
4. Cyanosis; patient's face and lips turn a blueish color.
5. Clonic phase; or the rapid, alternating contracting and relaxing of all the muscles of the body.
6. Breathing—may sound like snoring.
7. May lose control of bladder and bowels.
8. May bite the tongue resulting in blood stained saliva drooling from the mouth.
9. Gradual lessening of the spasm is followed by a period of unconsciousness. When the patient returns to consciousness he may be dazed and confused. Let him sleep if he wants to.
10. May complain of headache and sore muscles when he awakens.

Petit Mal

This is a "little" seizure and usually lasts from five to thirty seconds. There are three types of little seizures: in one, the patient simply stares, is unaware of what is going on and may go to sleep; in the second type, there are quick jerks of the head, arm or trunk muscles without any apparent loss of consciousness. When a patient has the third type, there is a sudden loss of control of the posture of the body, either falling to the ground or jackknifing his body on his legs.

Epileptic Equivalents

These are often called psychomotor attacks and are mental states in which there are disturbances of consciousness but no actual convulsion. The patient may appear dazed and unaware of what he is doing, may run a short distance, may become irritable or even violent, then return to his former behavior as though there had been no interruption.

Status Epilepticus

This is a complication of epilepsy in which seizures of any kind occur at frequent intervals and the patient remains unconscious in the period between seizures.

Jacksonian Epilepsy

This type is due to brain injury and there may not always be loss of consciousness. The seizure involves a limited group of muscles, depending upon the area of the brain that is injured. It may involve just the side of the face, or it may involve the entire one side of the body. The head and eyes are turned to the affected side.

Patients having epilepsy do not have a normal rhythm of brain waves. A special machine is used to make this test, which results in a tracing on paper called an electroencephalograph. This in turn can be used by the doctor to aid him in making a diagnosis of either idiopathic, or true, epilepsy and the type known as functional epilepsy. Some of the differences of behavior which the psychiatric technician can observe are:

SEIZURES

Idiopathic	*Functional*
More common among males	More frequent among females
Occurs night or day	Never occurs during sleep
Occurs any place	Occurs only when someone is nearby
Pupils of eyes inactive	Pupils of eyes active
Tongue may be bitten	Does not bite tongue, may chew lips
Cry out during aura; before fall	Cry out during seizure
Injuries frequent	Avoids hurting self
Movements typical	Movements not typical, may be sexually suggestive
Loses control of bladder and sometimes of bowels	Never loses control of bladder or bowels
Loss of consciousness	Aware of what goes on about them

WHAT THE PSYCHIATRIC TECHNICIAN CAN DO

A patient having any type of seizure needs care and attention. What you should do:

1. Keep calm; other patients tend to become unnecessarily upset if the nursing personnel get excited.
2. If you recognize the warning signals you may get to the patient before he falls and you can ease him to the floor.
3. Protect the head from injury by putting a pillow, a blanket, a coat or a jacket under it.
4. An object that cannot be swallowed, such as a soft mouth gag, a folded handkerchief, a tongue blade, a spoon handle

covered with a handkerchief or a piece of cloth of any kind, should be placed between the teeth on one side of the patient's mouth. This will aid in preventing damage to the teeth and will keep the patient from biting his tongue.

5. Do not force the object between the teeth; wait until the mouth opens, then insert the gag.

6. Loosen any clothing which may tend to be tight around the throat or waist.

7. Turn the head to one side if possible; this will aid in clearing the mouth of mucus and saliva.

8. Remain with the patient until the convulsing movements have stopped, then move him to his bed where he can sleep. He may need a bath and clean clothing if he lost control of his bladder and bowels during the seizure.

9. If a patient fails to regain consciousness before having another seizure, you may hear this spoken of as "going into status." The doctor should be called immediately. He may have to give the patient medicine by vein in order to bring the seizures under control.

GENERAL PRINCIPLES TO KEEP IN MIND

1. All patients who are subject to having seizures, do best if they have a regular schedule for all daily activities: personal hygiene, work and play.

2. They should eat the diet which has been ordered for them.

3. These patients must never be left alone at bath time.

4. They should not be permitted to participate in any activity which would endanger their life if they should have an unexpected seizure. For example, they should not be allowed to climb ladders.

5. Excessive fatigue should be avoided but plenty of exercise and fresh air are very beneficial for these patients.

6. Many drugs are used in the control of seizures, the specific ones being ordered by the doctor. If the psychiatric technician is held responsible for giving of medicines, it is especially important that the drugs for controlling seizures be given exactly as ordered both as to amount and time. Some

of the more common types of medicines ordered are dilantin and phenobarbital, in various dosages, for the control of grand mal type of seizure; tridione for the petit mal type and mesantoin for the Jacksonian type of seizure.

Chapter IV

CARING FOR THE PATIENT

THE WARD—STAGE FOR THERAPY

The ward, be it large or small, is the patient's home in the hospital. The furnishings of the ward play a very important part in the total treatment program of patients, just as do the personalities of the nursing staff.

As a psychiatric technician you may have worked on wards where the general atmosphere was tense and unpleasant, making you feel ill-at-ease and insecure as to your assignment. On other wards the atmosphere was congenial and relaxed, making it a real pleasure to have the assignment. Patients are extremely sensitive to the feeling of the ward environment. As a mentally ill patient whose work assignment was to help me in the office once said, "The vibrations aren't right, I can't work in there this morning," and returned to her home ward. Of course, this could have many interpretations, but on that particular morning there *was* a feeling of tenseness among the staff members due to a minor disagreement about assignments.

Materials for decorating, furniture, wall paints, floor finishes, and the physical layout of wards varies greatly among institutions. The old tradition was to have everything uniform and arranged to conform to a set standard, with great expanses of brown paint, plus large quantities of brown soap to keep everything clean.

The modern trend is to color, all shades and in many combinations, from the walls in the dayrooms to the beds in the dormitories. And what real harm is there in having the chairs in the living area "out-of-line" once in awhile? What kind of home do you have if you can't go to your bed for a nap when you want to be alone, to relax, for a little while?

Temperature and Ventilation

The best way to prevent unpleasant hospital odors is to have proper ventilation and to keep things clean by the vigorous use of cleansing agents (most of which have detergent action), water and elbow grease. Fresh air, without drafts, is good for all wards. It is sometimes difficult to adjust the temperature of the various ward areas to meet the needs of all patients. What is considered normal during the day will vary somewhat, but the average temperature is 68° to 72°. For very young children, the physically ill and the elderly patient the temperature should be a little higher, ranging from 75° to 80°. The average temperature for the night hours and best for sleeping, for most patients, is 65°.

Day or Living Room Areas

The furniture is usually selected according to the needs of the patients. Many patients can learn how to help care for furniture as well as other housekeeping duties. Other than the basic chairs and tables which are standard, many hospitals provide for television sets, radios, pianos and upholstered furniture, as well as lamps, books, magazines and window drapes for the ward day-rooms. Where the patients tend to be destructive, the window "drapes" can be in the form of a valance or as half curtains.

Some patients are quite clever at making small rugs and get real pleasure from seeing them used on their ward. However, small "throw" rugs do create a safety hazard and should not be used in the line of daily "traffic."

Patients' works of art such as finger paintings or crayon drawings can be used to decorate the ward. This in turn is therapeutic for the patient artist.

Growing plants and flowers in pots or other containers can be developed into an educational project for the patients. An example of a very inexpensive way to secure a beautiful growing vine for a ward living room is to place a medium sized sweet potato in a jar or can of water and just let it grow! Where such pets are permitted, patients can be taught to have the responsibility of caring for goldfish or a bird, such as a canary or a parakeet.

Dormitories or Sleeping Areas

Most ambulatory patients can learn how to make their own

beds and to keep their bedside cabinet, where provided, neat and clean. Girls like to keep a doll or other toy on their bed which adds a touch of extra color to a dormitory.

Weekly airing of the beds and change of linens should be routine.

Lavatory, Washroom, Toilet Areas

Absolute cleanliness is necessary to prevent odors. Ideally, there should be provision for a measure of privacy for the patient who must use the toilet.

Dining Rooms

Whether it be a dining area for patients from one ward or one which accommodates patients from several wards, it should be made as pleasant and cheerful as possible. This can be done by the addition of a bouquet of flowers on each table, either live cut flowers or a bunch of inexpensive plastic flowers. The latter are so easy to maintain and will last almost indefinitely. The use of other modern, colorful plastic products such as dishes, trays and curtains for the windows all aid in creating a therapeutic atmosphere. Where feasible, appropriate music creates an atmosphere of happy relaxation which contributes to a more complete enjoyment of the mealtime period.

Windows and doors should be screened to prevent the entry of flies. Kitchen and dining room areas are also prone to infestation with ants and cockroaches. Absolute cleanliness in all areas where food is prepared and served is the best preventive for this type of invasion. However, there are various commercial products available for use in the control of the various types of insects. Most institutions have their own method of controlling insects.

There are many other areas of a ward which must be kept clean, in order and repair, with observation of safety precautions at all times.

To paraphrase the words of the poet, it takes a heap of work to make a ward a home, but it can be done.

INTRODUCTION

Social custom decrees that an individual must conform to an established pattern of behavior: You wear a prescribed amount of clothing, you eat food at specified times and places, you bathe, brush your teeth and comb your hair at designated intervals, you work and play on a definite schedule, and you never urinate or defecate in public.

The mentally retarded patient requires intensive training to enable him to fit into this cultural pattern and the amount of time required will vary with the degree of retardation of the child. Any person who is to achieve satisfaction in working with retarded children must always bear in mind that it takes time, months and years of time; and patience, an infinite amount of patience.

The responsibility for establishing and maintaining a habit training program falls upon the nursing personnel in a hospital; in the majority of hospitals this means the psychiatric technician. He must be able to accept the patient as he is, each as an individual that has some characteristic that sets him apart from the others. The relationship between the psychiatric technician and the patient is a close one, in most instances extending over a period of years. For many patients, the chief medicine which they receive is the attention and care given them by the technicians.

A carefully planned and executed routine is a necessity when training patients in socially acceptable behavior. As a psychiatric technician once said, it takes all of your time, just feeding one end, then cleaning the other. The technician must have flexibility to adjust to the demands of large numbers of children as well as an endless amount of patience if he is to cope with the multitude of problems associated with the feeding and toileting of severely retarded patients.

DISCIPLINE

It is neither kind nor fair to a child, be he normal or retarded, if he is spared discipline and is not required to learn socially acceptable behavior. A brief description of the word "discipline" which should be kept in mind when working with retarded children is: "training which corrects, molds, strengthens or perfects."* All nursing personnel need to have a basic knowledge of fundamen-

---

*Webster's New Collegiate Dictionary, Springfield, Mass., G. & C. Merriam Co., publishers of the Merriam-Webster Dictionaries, 1961, p. 236.

tals of establishing discipline and this can be summarized by the
*ABC's of Good Discipline.**

A. for affection; a basic tie between any teacher and pupil.
B. for balance; or a wise weighing of values.
C. for consistency; of goals, not always methods, and tempered by the
    individual differences of place and time.
D. for democracy; or the rights of the individual to self-respect and a
    feeling of personal worth.
E. for effort, which must be continuous and never ceasing.
F. for firmness; this does not mean rigidity.
G. for generosity, of both your time and patience.
H. for helpfulness, ever-ready and wisely given.
I. for imagination, in finding new and better ways of doing the job.
J. for joyousness; the delights of success should be every day.
K. for kindness, at all times.
L. for laughter, the balance wheel in times of stress.
M. for management; the wise choice of methods.
N. for nature; of good health in emotional relationships.
O. for outlets, or direction of drives into ways acceptable.
P. for praise, never stinted.
Q. for quietness; frequent freedom from anxieties and excitements.
R. for routine, necessary and comfortable.
S. for security; safety and protection from unnecessary dangers.
T. for tolerance, of failure and weaknesses.
U. for understanding, of individual differences in interests and skills.
V. for vigilance; watchfulness for danger signals.
W. for warmth; or the readiness to express affection.
X. to mark the place—here and now.
Y. for "Yeses"—may they outnumber the "No's."
Z. for Zest for today and tomorrow.

TOILET TRAINING

The teaching of this "habit" is, perhaps more than any other,
dependent upon a set time schedule. Be a *"clock-watcher!"* Whether

---

*Blodgett, Harriett E. and Warfield, Grace J.: *Understanding Mentally Re-
tarded Children,* New York, Appleton-Century-Crofts, 1959, p. 100.

it be every hour, every two or every four hours, it must be consistently followed through by all shifts on a ward.

An all-important factor upon which hinges a successful toilet training regime is the attitude of a person working with the patients. An individual who is repulsed and disgusted at the sight of a feces-smeared child should not try to work with severely retarded patients. Neither can a person work successfully with them if he is easily disturbed and upset when a routine does not always conform with what the "book says."

Unorthodox as it may sound, toilet-training can be a "socializing" time. By this is meant that not only does the employee talk and explain all procedures to the patients, no matter how retarded

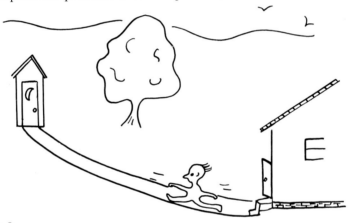

Figure 9.
    Jack be nimble
    Be emphatic
    Potting training
    Can be traumatic

they may be, but by working with small groups, the patients learn by watching and imitating others. Toilet time should be one of relaxation, not one of haste and anxiety. Psychologically, to most people, elimination of waste is a pleasurable idea. It should not be made a fearful or "disgusting" process.

Directions which are helpful in establishing a routine are:
1. Take the child to the toilet
    a. On rising.
    b. Before and after each meal.

    c. At his bedtime.

    d. Awake him fully later in the evening, always at the same hours, and take or have him go, to the toilet.

2. Serve the evening meal at a regular time.

    a. Reduce the liquid intake after the evening meal, unless there are medical contraindications.

Things to Avoid

1. Considering soiling and wetting as something that cannot be corrected.
2. Discouraging the patient in any way.
3. Making the patient feel ashamed.
4. Spending a long time in the bathroom.
5. Playing with toys while on the toilet.
6. Making the excuse of sickness when patient is really well.
7. Scolding. It is useless and often times harmful.

Helpful Hints

1. Children like praise! Reward success with praise.
2. Children like to do what is expected of them and you will get about what you expect of them.
3. Large buttons and easily handled clothing, such as training panties, will enable the patient to help himself more easily.
4. Toilet facilities to meet the age and size of the patient are of great assistance in training a child to use the toilet.

    a. Toilet seats on the toilet aid the child in overcoming his fear of falling into the water.

REGULARITY

A carefully planned, regular routine to cover the hourly activities in a twenty-four hour period is a necessity in teaching a retarded patient socially acceptable behavior. It means, as far as is possible, doing the same thing, in the same place, at the same time of day, week in and week out.

Emphasize one habit at a time and provide an opportunity for success; after all, everyone is happier if they get satisfaction out of what is being done. Remember that the attention span of a mentally retarded child is short and constant repetition is a necessity.

An example of a typical 24-hour schedule would be:

6:30	AM—Dormitory lights turned on.
6:40	—Instructions in dressing and bedmaking.
7:00	—Ward housekeeping.
7:15	—Prepare for breakfast—toilet drill.
7:45	—Breakfast.
8:15	—Toothbrush drill.
8:30	—Ward housekeeping.
8:45	—Personal grooming or beauty culture.
9:00	—Toilet drill.
9:00-10:00 AM	—Occupational Therapy.
10:00-11:15	—Recreational Therapy.
11:15	—Toilet drill—handwashing.
11:30	—Lunch
12:00 Noon	—Clean-up drill.
12:05	PM—Toothbrush drill.
12:30	PM—Free time.
1:00- 2:00	—Occupational Therapy.
2:00	—Toilet drill.
2:10- 3:00	—Walking.
3:00	—Clean-up drill—toilet routine.
4:00	—Supper.
4:45	—Toothbrush drill—personal hygiene.
5:00- 6:45	—Reading, games, TV, outdoor activities as climate permits, social activities.
6:45	—Toilet drill.
7:00	—Ward cleaning.
8:00	—Bedtime.
10:15	—Toileting—untidy, ambulatory patients— "Specialing" for bedfast patients.
1:00	AM—Toileting—untidy, ambulatory patients— "Specialing" for bedfast patients.
3:00	—Toileting—untidy, ambulatory patients— "Specialing" for bedfast patients.
5:00	—Toileting—untidy, ambulatory patients— "Specialing" for bedfast patients.

6:30   —Lights on, for the start of another day.

Don't become discouraged too soon when establishing a habit training program.

Remember

1. The retarded patient is not able, to any great degree, to use past experience to help him solve an immediate problem.
2. The retarded patient wants to conform.
3. A retarded patient needs firm, consistent handling by those who care for him.
4. Directions must be simple and specific.
5. Teaching by showing rather than by telling is more productive when working with the retarded patient.
6. The patient will not respond at once; repetition is a MUST.

Avoid

1. Confusing the issue with useless talk.
2. Lengthy or detailed directions.
3. Setting a goal too far in the future.
4. Having the patient wait too long for things he needs or wants.
5. Changes, unless made slowly.

NUTRITION AND THE EATING HABIT

The act of eating is, for most of us, done routinely three times a day without much thought about it; in fact it is a very pleasant habit. This is far from true for many patients, one of the greatest nursing care problems pertaining to the severely mentally retarded patient being that of maintaining an adequate intake of food.

Many retarded children have not progressed beyond the bottle feeding stage when admitted to a hospital, although physically there is no reason for them not to have learned how to eat. This may have been the result of the mother not knowing how to teach the child to eat, or she may have wanted to avoid a "messy" table, or she may have been over-protective toward the child.

Some patients when admitted to the hospital have never learned how to chew solid foods, even though there is nothing physically wrong, such as defective teeth.

All children should learn to eat and to feed themselves as early as possible and the change from bottle feeding to solid foods should be made as soon as it can be managed and still meet the nutritional needs of each child.

Bottle Feeding

A child normally should give up the bottle by the end of his first year; with the mentally retarded child it is not unusual to want and need the bottle for a much longer time. The "weaning" just has to take place a little later.

Ideally, the child should be held by the psychiatric technician while being given his bottle. However, in many hospital situations it is necessary to prop both the child and the bottle with pillows or small blankets at feeding times. Whether held by the Technician or propped on a pillow, the bottle should be in such a position that the nipple remains filled with milk, otherwise the child will suck air; the child should be "burped" during his feeding as this will help him bring up the air which he may have swallowed. This is usually done by holding the child over your shoulder and patting him gently on the back until he belches. When the feeding is finished the child should be "burped" again and placed on his right side in his bed. If the child's mouth is open when the nipple is removed, there will be less of a chance that some of the formula will be expelled into his mouth which might cause him to choke and perhaps vomit his feeding.

Self-feeding

Milk is a child's first food and should be a part of his regular diet throughout his life. After weaning, every child should have an adequate diet containing, besides milk, cereal and bread, fruits and vegetables, butter and eggs, and meat, cheese, fish and poultry.

The ability to handle a cup and spoon is acquired slowly and requires an endless amount of patience when training retarded patients. It may take six months or longer to teach one child to eat from a spoon, then more months to get him to hold the spoon for himself.

Normally this training can be started at about the age of four months. With the retarded patients the 4-month level may not be achieved for years! Individual capabilities have a wide range and must all be taken into consideration, with the exception of the severely retarded, extremely physically handicapped patients, all patients can be trained to eat in a socially acceptable manner. All ambulatory, as well as many wheelchair patients can be taught to take their place at the table in a dining room. Where cafeteria service is used, all ambulatory patients can be taught to pass by the counter, picking up their trays, utensils and food. Following their meal, they can also be taught how to return their tray and utensils to the designated place, before leaving the dining area.

Helpful Hints

1. Control of child's hands
   The technician must sit at the right side of the child, her left arm behind him, her left hand controlling his left hand. Her right hand is then free to guide the spoon in the child's right hand. If she sits opposite she can control neither of the child's hands. (This pertains to the child if he is sitting in a highchair or at a table.)

2. Practice in eating soft solid foods
   Place a small amount of thick food such as soaked cereal or mashed fruit on the tip of a shallow spoon or on the handle of a spoon. Have the child use his lips (not his teeth) to remove the food from the spoon. Do not let the spoon scrape against the upper teeth.

3. Practice in chewing
   Put a small amount of food in one side of the mouth toward the back. Feed from one side and then the other. Do not put the food in the center of the mouth. Tell the child to chew. Show him by moving your own jaw up and down. Then show him how to move his jaw up and down.

4. Swallowing
   Teach the child to move his jaws as little as possible when swallowing. Have the child feel his own throat when he swallows, so that he will become aware of the act of swallowing.

Try standing behind the child and holding his jaw in one hand while you hold the cup with the other.*

PRINCIPLES TO KEEP IN MIND WHEN FEEDING HANDICAPPED PATIENTS

1. Treat them as individuals.
   a. Stimulate his appetite by trying first the food he likes best on his tray.
   b. Thicken his beverage or cereal with bread crumbs if he can eat better by this means.
   c. Take care that the food is not too hot. Cool it with milk or bread crumbs or spread out on the tray.
   d. Get second helpings for him if he wants more.
2. Child must feel secure.
3. Child must feel comfortable, his position while being fed being important.
   a. If at all possible, bring him to the table and seat him in front of his tray.
   b. If spoon feeding is required, place him in the position best suited to his needs; upright, head slightly tilted back or chair tilted back.
4. Socialize with the patient while feeding him.
   a. In a hospital setting meal time is often times the only opportunity for the nursing person to sit down and talk to or with the patient.
5. Patients who do not eat well may learn by observing others.

Points to Remember at Meal Time

1. Try to maintain a calm, unworried attitude towards the childrens' eating.
2. Serve meals at regular time.
3. Make the food attractive and give small amounts in each serving.
   a. A big plateful of food set in front of child may discourage him from trying to eat.

---

*New Mexico Department of Public Health: Helpful Hints for the Child Who Does Not Eat or Swallow Easily, Pamphlet 103, Santa Fe, New Mexico, 1961.

   b. Small helpings will also discourage playing with the food and messing it up.
4. Try new foods a little at a time; try them more than once.
   a. Some children will accept only pureed types of foods and will choke on chopped foods; others will take only crisp, crunchy food. Sometimes they will delay as long as four or five years before they will accept any in-between foods.
5. Have the children understand that eating is the business at hand and that he is expected to eat it (the meal).
6. Refeed the food he spits out. This will help him to learn that it is good food.
7. Don'ts at Meal Time
   a. Feed the child if he is able to feed himself.
   b. Coax, threaten or force the child to eat.
   c. Talk about his likes or dislikes in front of him.
   d. Talk about his poor appetite in his hearing.
   e. Worry if the child misses a meal or two while learning to eat as others do.
   f. Deprive a child of a meal for punishment.

SPECIAL PROBLEMS

1. *Anorexia*, or lack or loss of appetite, will result in a patient refusing to eat a part of or even all food offered him. There are numerous reasons why this occurs: it may be only temporary when a child is cutting teeth, it may be due to an emotional upset, it may be due to a feeling of frustration because life hasn't gone the way the person wanted it to, or there may be no apparent reason of any kind. If the patient cannot be persuaded to take nourishment by spoon-feeding, the special procedure of tube-feeding (passing a tube through the mouth or nose, down the throat and into the stomach) must be used. This procedure is done by a doctor or a registered nurse.

2. *Regurgitation* is the process of food being expelled without force from the patient's stomach (vomiting is the forceful expulsion of food) following his feeding. It will seem as though the food simply flows backward. The cause for this is not always easily determined but it is important to know when it occurs and the kind

of food that is not retained. Some patients will retain solids
but not liquids and vice versa. Some patients will regurgitate if
held after feeding instead of being placed immediately in their
bed. Prevention must be determined by the individual patient's
needs.

3. Self-induced regurgitation with a chewing and reswallowing of
the food is called *rumination*. The most common method of in-
ducing regurgitation is by the patient to put his finger, or fingers, down his throat. Sometimes a patient can do this by swallowing air or there may be no apparent reason for it to occur.
Rumination may occur for a short time following the addition
of new foods to the diet. Measures which can be taken to prevent rumination include distraction of the child's attention immediately following his feeding, change the feeding schedule or
a mild form of arm restraint is helpful with some patients.

4. *The Blind Patient*. The child who has never had sight must learn
to feed himself and to use the spoon and other utensils by the
sense of touch. To help him learn about foods, the psychiatric
technician should give a colorful description and the name of
each item, and repeat the name of the food each time it is served.
When feeding a blind child he should be told whether it is going
to be hot or cold. When assisting a patient who is temporarily
blind, such as following some types of treatments, the same methods would apply.

5. *The Cerebral Palsy Patient*. Assuring an adequate intake of food
for this type of patient is a real nursing care challenge. The
athetoid type presents the major problem because they not only
have an almost continuous movement of the fingers and toes
but also have spasms of the muscles of swallowing and breathing.
They frequently gag during the feeding because the tongue is
"swallowed." Many times the movement of the tongue reverses
and this interferes with the swallowing of food. When spoon-feeding such a child, the food should be placed well back on the
tongue, with an unhurried, steady rate and with a relaxed manner on the part of the technician.

When teaching a child to feed himself special equipment may be
available, or simple modifications of regular equipment can be
devised.

TOOLS FOR EATING

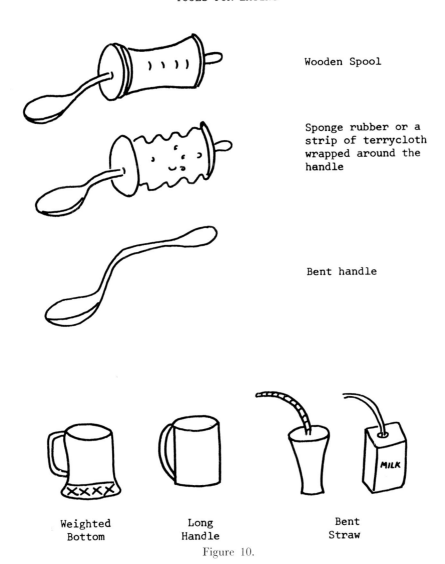

Wooden Spool

Sponge rubber or a
strip of terrycloth
wrapped around the
handle

Bent handle

Weighted Bottom   Long Handle   Bent Straw

Figure 10.

A BONUS SUGGESTION

There are many patients who cannot participate at meal time in a conventional type of dining room setting because of the structure of the chairs and tables.

A table surface, in the form of a lapboard, may be used for patients who must remain in a wheelchair or a chair with armrests. The board rests on the arms of the chair and extends over the sides and front. Cloth straps may be threaded through the holes near the back of the board and tie around the chair to hold the board in place. The size of the patient, the chair and the amount of surface will determine the dimensions of the board. The inner edge of the board should rest close to the patient; the width and depth

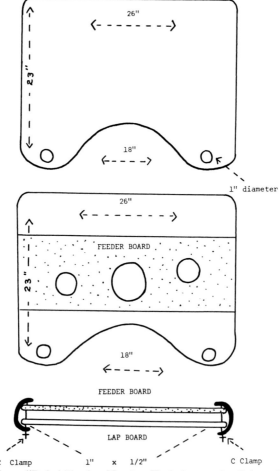

Figure 11. From "Rehabilitative Nursing Techniques—2: Selected Equipment Useful in the Hospital, Home, or Nursing Home," Minneapolis: Kenny Rehabilitation, 1962, by permission from the publisher.

of the cut-out may have to be adjusted for a very large or a very small patient.

For the patient who lacks coordination or who is unable to handle his own eating equipment, a *feeder attachment* may be added to the lapboard. Both the lapboard and the attachment may be made out of plywood. The holes in the attachment are cut through the wood to fit the dishes, cups and glasses that the patient will be using. They should be so placed to enable him to reach the articles easily. A suggested adult size is shown in Figure 11.

DISEASES WHICH MAY RESULT FROM MALNUTRITION

1. Anemia, primary or secondary—due to lack of iron in the diet.
2. Beriberi—due to lack of vitamin B1 in the diet.
3. Pellegra—due to lack of niacin in the diet.
4. Rickets—due to lack of vitamin D, calcium and phosphorus in the diet.
5. Scurvy—due to lack of vitamin C in the diet.
6. Simple goitre—due to lack of iodine.

TYPES OF DIETS

Diets served in hospitals vary and to a great extent depend upon not only the institution but also upon its geographical location. Standard diets which may be modified to meet many needs are:

1. Regular—normal diet which each day contains the correct proportion of protein, carbohydrates, fats, minerals, vitamins, roughage and water.
2. Soft—bland (not highly seasoned) foods which are low in roughage.
3. Full liquid—milk drinks, fruit juices, gelatin, plain ice cream, strained soups and gruel, tea, coffee and carbonated beverages.
4. Clear liquid—strained fruit juices, broth, tea, coffee and carbonated beverages.
5. Special diets—ordered individually by the doctor.

BASIC NURSING CARE

Mentally retarded patients have physical illnesses just as normal people do. Many of them when sick, will be in pain, be frightened and anxious but will not be able to express themselves or be able to tell how they feel. Do not ignore them—while it is not the technician's duty to diagnose a patient's ailment, it is his duty to be alert at all times to the physical condition of the patients entrusted to his care. Early recognition of physical ills is usually dependent upon the skilled observation of the technician who must report anything unusual immediately to the doctor. The doctor will want to know among other things, if the patient has an elevated temperature, or fever, and his pulse and respiration.

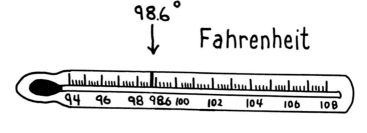

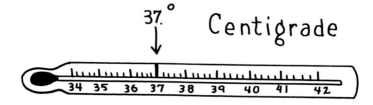

Clinical Thermometers
Figure 12.

TEMPERATURE, PULSE AND RESPIRATION

A clinical thermometer, either oral (by mouth) or rectal (by rectum) is used to measure the heat of the body, or temperature.

Normal temperature by mouth is 98.6 degrees by a Fahrenheit (F) thermometer or 99.6 degrees by rectum. A moderate fever would range from 100° F to 103° F. There are two types of thermometers in use, the "Centigrade" and the "Fahrenheit." On the Centigrade the lowest mark is "0" degrees, written as 0° C and the highest mark is 100° C, the distance between 0 and 100 being divided into 100 equal degrees. The lowest mark on the Fahrenheit thermometer is 32 degrees, written as 32° F, the highest mark is 212° F. The distance between these two points is divided into 180 equal degrees.

The pulse is the beat of the heart as it pumps the blood into the blood vessels. The pulse can be taken anywhere an artery is close to the surface of the skin, the most common place being the radial artery, or the artery that crosses the bone on the thumb side of the

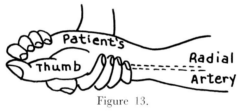

Figure 13.

wrist. When taking a pulse, place the tips of the first three fingers of your hand over the artery, using only enough pressure to feel the "beat." Do not put your thumb over the artery as you will feel your own pulse. Average rates for one minute for an infant are 110-130; for children 1-7 years of age, 80-120; for children over 7 years, 72-90; for women, 65 to 80 and for men, 60 to 70.

The respiration is the breathing of a patient, a complete respiration being the drawing into the lungs and the letting out, of one breath of air. Average rates for one minute for an infant are 30 to 35; for children, 20 to 35; for women, 18 to 20; and for men, 16 to 18.

BATHING AND CARE OF THE SKIN

1. *Babies* must be bathed as often as necessary to keep them clean, dry and skin in good condition. Any time the baby is soiled with feces or urine he must be bathed with a mild soap and water,

not just wiped off with one end of the diaper. After washing, the skin must be thoroughly dried and may be dusted with powder. Babies may be bathed in their cribs; the use of slab tubs greatly facilitate the bathing procedure be it an infant or an adult who is handicapped and infirm. When giving the daily bath, special attention must be given to the ears, nose and areas around the eyes. The bathroom should be without drafts, and warm, with all bathing supplies in a convenient place. An individual wash cloth and towel must be used for each patient. The temperature of the bath water should be 99° to 105° F, never beyond 105°F. The temperature should be checked with a bath thermometer; if one is not available, test the water by letting some run on the inner surface of your arm.

Special Precautions

1. When diapering, or performing a nursing procedure, do not leave the child alone.

2. Keep one hand on the child when reaching for any article.

3. Do not leave safety pins lying about as the baby may put them in his mouth.

4. Be sure the crib sides are securely fastened before leaving the child.

2. *Severely retarded, extremely physically handicapped patients* require total nursing care. The hydrocephalic and the spastic type patients require constant, special attention to their skin to prevent the development of bedsores (decubitis ulcers). Bedsores result when there is an interference in the circulation in a part of the body, which may be due to pressure, lying too long in one position or by splints, casts, or weight of bedclothes. The condition is further aggravated by neglect in cleaning the patient following soiling with feces or urine, perspiration or other moisture, wrinkles in the bedclothes or crumbs left in the bed following a meal. A bedsore is almost without exception preventable, and it is usually due to careless nursing if one develops. Warning signs are heat, redness, tenderness and discomfort in the area.

Prevention

Keep patient and bed clean and dry.

Keep bed free from wrinkles and crumbs.

Change patient's position frequently, every 2 to 3 hours.

Give special skin care such as an alcohol rub, followed by dusting with a talcum powder.

Pressure may be eased or avoided by using:

  a. Rubber air rings under bony parts, such as the ankles, elbows, heels.

  b. Pad and gauze bandage.

  c. Small pillows.

  d. Air mattress or air pillows.

  e. *Sheepskin* or *synthetic fiber pads,* used under bony prominences, such as the heels and elbows, and under the head of a hydrocephalic patient, are very helpful in the prevention of decubitus ulcers.

There is always a lot of lifting involved in caring for the infirm patient; it is therefore, important for the psychiatric technician to know how to lift and move patients so as to cause as little discomfort as possible. A knowledge of correct body mechanics will also aid in preventing undue strain and fatigue for yourself.

Ten rules for lifting which you should keep in mind and practice are:

  1. Size up the load.

  2. Face the load squarely.

  3. Never lift from a kneeling position.

  4. Bend your knees.

  5. Get a good grip on the load.

  6. Keep a straight back and lift by straightening your legs.

  7. Lift slowly and evenly.

  8. Keep the load close to your body.

  9. Don't twist your body.

  10. In "team lifting" let only one man give the signals and then lift together.

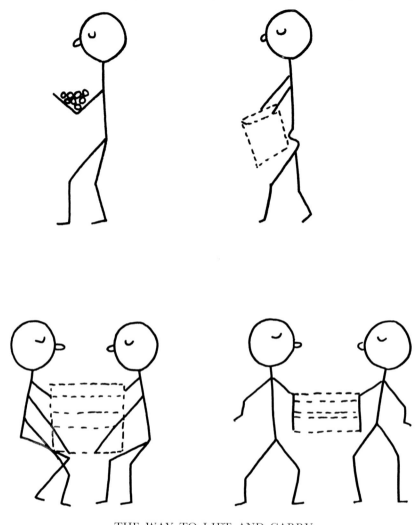

THE WAY TO LIFT AND CARRY

Figure 14. Smaller loads are best carried in your arms with the weight close to your body and the shoulders bent.

Figure 15. Heavier weights of smaller size are best carried with a straight back and arms and placed somewhat to one side (i.e., on the hip).

Figure 16. The double lift: Don't lift or carry a weight for two men alone—get help. For a double lift, that is when two people are going to lift a weight together, they must always move together. The same is true when two people carry a weight.

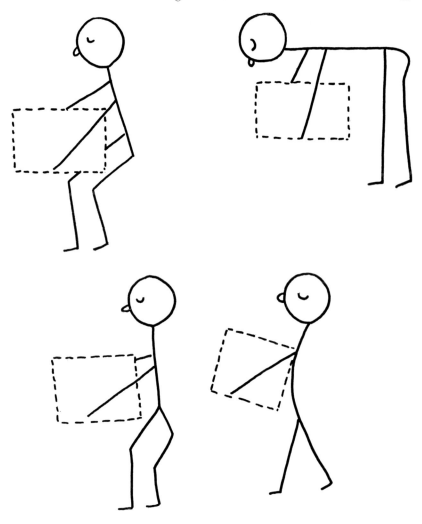

Figure 17. *Right.* Straight arms, straight back. The muscle work is done mainly by the thigh and buttock muscles.

Figure 18. *Wrong.* The back is bent far forward and legs straight. This is a strain for the back.

Figure 19. Lift and carry in a labor saving way. If you want to lift a heavy weight from table height you should stand close to the table with your legs slightly bent and arms straight. Then grasp the weight directly, place it against the body and lift, at the same time stretching the legs and leaning the body back. Don't sway too much.

3. *Ambulatory* patients may be given their bath in a tub or shower. The bathroom must be warm and free from drafts. When giving a tub bath remember to use less water for a child than for an adult. No patient should be permitted to remain in the tub longer than 10 or 15 minutes without a doctor's orders, and the patient should always be supervised by an employee. If you find that you cannot assist the patient out of the tub by yourself, let the water run out of the tub, protect the patient with a towel or bath blanket and call for assistance.

The temperature of the water for a shower bath should be regulated *before* the patient enters the shower. Shower caps should be provided for girls and women. If the shower is not equipped with a hand rail, it is helpful to have a stool or straight chair available for the use of patients who are unsteady on their feet. It is important to protect the patient from unnecessary exposure during the bathing procedure by use of screens and the provision of robes, or clothing, to wear to and from the bathroom.

The actual number of baths given a patient per week will depend upon many factors, but suggested minimums are:

1. Bed patients—daily bath.
2. Incontinent (lack of control of bladder or bowels)—bathe whenever necessary.
3. Ambulatory patients—3 baths or showers per week.
4. Working patients—daily shower or bath.

Bath time is the opportunity to make careful check of the patients' entire body and specifically the skin, nails and scalp. Trimming of toenails and fingernails may be done best following the

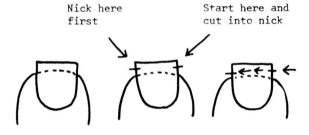

TRIMMING TOENAILS
Figure 20.

bath. Toenails should be cut straight across. In order to prevent breakage of thin or brittle nails, one should make a cut on one side of the nail. then start from the other side. Deformed, ingrown or injured nails should be referred to the ward doctor. Athlete's foot is a very common fungus infection of the skin of feet and of the areas between the toes. One of the best preventive measures is *thorough drying* of the areas between toes following daily bathing of the feet.

4. Special Skin Care

Many of the mentally retarded patients have sensitive skin that chaps and/or sunburns easily. The mildest of soaps sometimes will prove to be irritating to their skin. It is usually permissible to apply a cold cream, vaseline or a baby oil to the patient's skin if such conditions occur. Specific orders are obtained from the doctor. Many of the patients have frequent colds and runny noses. To prevent sores and irritations of the skin about the nose and face from developing, noses must be kept clean.

1. Teach patients to blow and clean their noses.
2. Use squares of toilet tissue if handkerchiefs or kleenex are unavailable.

The patients' eyes may become slightly irritated and crusts develop around the lids.

1. Wash frequently with warm water. This not only makes the patient more comfortable but reduces the possibility of a more serious condition developing.
2. Special eye ointments may be applied if ordered by the ward doctor.

PREVENTION OF DEFORMITIES

Many mentally retarded patients have the additional handicap of physical disabilities, some being of a congenital nature (born with); others being acquired as a result of inadequate nursing care. The elderly, or geriatric, patient is also prone to the development of deformities due to inactivity or improper bed positioning. In fact, any patient regardless of his diagnosis, may develop varying degrees and types of deformities if he:

1. Is confined to bed for a long period of time.
2. Sits in a wheelchair for many hours at a time.
3. Is permitted to remain in one position too long at a time.
4. Is not given corrective exercises.

Deformity prevention and active physical therapy treatment require trained physical therapists, but a *control* program can be carried on by ward nursing personnel who have been taught by a physical therapist.

Nursing care problems are reduced if patients function at their maximum; for example, a patient who can walk on straight legs is easier to care for than who cannot walk due to contractures of the limbs. Goals for motor function are variable and not the same for all patients, just as growth and development patterns differ.

The use of physical therapy techniques at ward level consist basically of good bedside nursing procedures. The extent to which "physical therapy" is performed by ward nursing personnel will depend upon the institution. However, nursing care revolves around the daily activities of the patient: bathing, personnel hygiene in and out of bed, up and down from a chair and in the use of various toilet facilities. During the process of giving the daily bath it is possible, for example, to exercise most of the patient's muscles and joints. If the patient remains in bed, correct positioning can be accomplished by the use of various types of supports. Appropriate change of position should be done at regular intervals. Correct position with the appropriate variations should also be carried out for the patient who spends many hours in a wheelchair.

Supportive devices such as pillows, blanket or towel rolls, sandbags, air cushions, foam rubber pads and footboards may be used to relieve pressure. Materials which are readily available can be utilized for many purposes; for example, two washcloths rolled firmly together and fastened with tape can be used as a handroll. Many times one or both hands of a patient may be flexed (semi-fist like position) and if allowed to remain this way will become permanently deformed. This is not only painful for the patient and difficult to keep clean but without the full use of his thumb, the patient will have difficulty in manipulating buttons and buttonholes as well as having problems in turning a doorknob and other daily activities. The handroll is used to aid in maintaining the functional position of the hand; that is, bringing the thumb and forefinger opposite to each other.

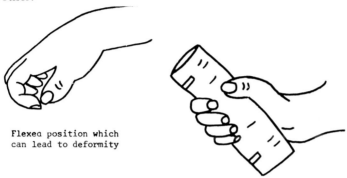

Flexea position which
can lead to deformity

Position of a handroll

Figure 21

A footboard may be used to maintain the correct position of the feet of a patient who is confined to bed for a long time.

Specific types of exercise may be utilized by nursing personnel following instruction from a physical therapist and upon the physician's orders. Exercise may be of various types, all designed for the purpose of maintaining flexibility and the prevention of contractures. The processes of exercising also stimulate the circulation, increase appetite and enhance the sense of well-being of the patient.

"Massage," which is defined as the scientific manipulation of the soft tissue of the body, has a great psychological effect on a patient. The physical "laying on of hands" has a reassuring value and the patient enjoys the personal attention given him. Methods of relaxation followed by careful muscle re-education should ultimately result in the patient being able to care for himself up to the limits of his ability.

Patients, with very few exceptions, or as ordered by the ward physician, should not be permitted to remain flat on their back 24 hours a day. They should be given the opportunity to learn how to crawl or creep, by putting them on a blanket on the floor, before expecting them to learn how to walk. If this is not practical or expedient, the patient should be gotten up and into a wheelchair, walker or stroller, or similar device. If there is no wheelchair available, place any type of chair which has arms by the side of the bed and get the patient out of bed and into it for a change of position.

Nursing personnel who aid in the rehabilitation of patients should find the following directions of assistance.

THE PRINCIPLES OF EXERCISE*

1. Contract the muscles as hard as possible.
   a. The amount of motion obtained is of secondary importance.
   b. Full power contraction squeezes the blood out of the tissue, carrying away the products of fatigue. Actual tension of the muscle tissue is necessary to produce this pumping action.
2. Relax completely while you take at least two deep breaths.
   a. Relaxation allows the blood to flow back to the part to nourish the tissue.
3. Do not hold your breath in order to augment muscular effort.
   a. Holding your breath markedly increases the rapidity and extent of fatigue.
   b. Relaxation of the rest of the body is necessary to obtain maximum effort with minimal fatigue.
4. Concentrate on what you are doing and take time to do it right.
   a. Exercises done at double time and half power are a waste of time.
5. The effect of therapeutic exercises (increased nourishment to the tissue) lasts about 4 hours.
   a. Exercises for short periods (three to ten minutes) several times a day are necessary to alleviate pain from muscular tension and to build up muscle tone, (twenty minutes once a day will not substitute for five minutes four times a day).
6. Muscle tension can build up from many causes.
   a. Muscle tension can be improved by increasing the circulation to the part with therapeutic exercise but only if the exercise is done properly, i.e., not beyond the point of fatigue and frequently enough to keep the circulation adequate.

ORAL HYGIENE

The mouth and teeth of every patient should be cleansed a

Orthopedic Nursing Procedures. Avice Kerr, R.N., B.A., Springer Publishing Co., Inc., N. Y., N. Y., pp. 299-300, by permission of the author and the publisher.

minimum of once daily, preferably after every meal, not only for hygiene reasons but to prevent decaying of the teeth.

Many patients can be taught to brush their own teeth and with persistent practice can do it satisfactorily. Brushing not only cleans the teeth but hardens the gums. There are many opinions as to how teeth are brushed but the procedure should include both the teeth and gums. A commonly accepted method is to brush *down-*

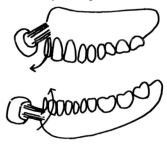

ward on the upper teeth and *upward* on the lower ones, on both the inside and the outside. Brushing across sometimes actually forces food particles deeper into the spaces between the teeth. A piece of dental floss may be used to remove food particles which become wedged between two teeth. The only place that should be brushed *across* is when the tops of the lower and the bottom of the upper,

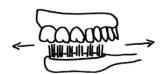

back teeth or molars are cleaned. Care should be taken not to injure the gum tissue. The use of electric toothbrushes has been reported as being quite helpful in carrying out the procedure on uncooperative patients, as well as being very beneficial in promoting healing of the gums. The entire procedure should always be under the supervision of the psychiatric technician. Every patient must have his own toothbrush.

The type of mouth washes and tooth pastes used will vary with the hospital and with the individual. Satisfactory and inexpensive substitutes for the commercial preparations are common table salt and baking soda.

Patients who wear dentures may need close supervision in both the wearing of and the proper cleansing of the dentures.

Patients who are given certain medicines for the control of seizures will sometimes develop soft, spongy gums which tend to bleed easily when the teeth are brushed. This must be called to the doctor's attention as the toothbrushing should not be neglected.

Special mouth care must be given to the severely retarded and physically handicapped patients: An applicator dipped in a mouthwash solution is used to clean the inside of the mouth, the teeth, tongue and roof of the mouth. A tongue blade may be used to aid in holding the mouth open.

The mouths of patients who are "mouth-breathers" are prone to become dry and the tongue "coated." It is usually permissible to use a solution composed of four parts of mineral oil to one part of lemon juice to moisten the lips and mouth of such patients.

Dentists usually recommend that an individual have a dental examination at least every six months. However, there is no substitute for good oral hygiene.

MENSTRUATION

With the onset of puberty, the monthly menstrual period will occur with female patients. The actual age and the establishment of regularity of the monthly cycle will vary greatly among retarded patients. The female psychiatric technician, as the "substitute mother" must explain this occurrence to the patient in the way best adapted to the patient's ability to understand. Some patients do not have the mental ability to understand why a sanitary napkin should be worn nor how to care for themselves. It is the technician's responsibility to give the required personal hygiene to prevent embarrassment to the patient and to those around her.

Many times changes occur in a patient's behavior which are related to the menstrual cycle. The behavior may vary from a state of increased irritability, or a mild depression or even a state of mild excitement and hyperactivity. If a record is kept of these variations in behavior it will serve as a guide for you as to how to manage the patient during these periods because each patient will have her own individual behavior pattern.

It is also advisable to keep a catamenial (menses) chart for each female patient, indicating the dates on which the menstrual period began and when it ended.

CLOTHES AND LEARNING HOW TO DRESS

Attractive, neat and appropriate clothing is a necessity in teaching retarded patients good grooming and to take pride in their personal appearance. Clothing should not be elaborate nor does it need to be expensive. Simple styles, in attractive colors and of serviceable wash materials are best. All garments should be easy to get on and off, with fasteners that are easy to manipulate. A tape fastener made from Velcro or similar type material is easier to manage than zipper or button fronts. (Velcro tape strips lock together when they come into contact with each other; it requires only a light touch and can be opened by simply pulling apart.)

Most hospitals and schools provide garments of a special type of heavy material for destructive patients and it is therapeutically desirable for this too to be colorful as well as "strong."

In most state facilities, parents or responsible persons are encouraged to provide clothing for their children.

All clothing should be individually fitted for a patient; sometimes this can be achieved by the use of a belt or an elastic waist band in dresses for the girls and in the boxer jeans or trousers for the boys. Little extra touches mean a lot not only to little folks but to the older ones as well. A colorful ribbon for a girl's hair, or a tie or belt for a boy, will do much to lift their spirits. If a child has difficulty in learning how to tell front from back, a bright colored tab, pocket or fake patch can be sewed on the garment in an appropriate place.

Special attention should be given to the fit and type of clothing which is worn by patients who spend many hours in a wheelchair. Unnecessary bulk should be avoided as it can cause the individual to become very uncomfortable.

All patients should be taught the importance of having clean underwear and be provided the opportunity to change if necessary.

Cotton knit panties for girls are more practical than the rayon or nylon type. For the female patient who has difficulty in fastening her brassiere the back opening can be converted to a front opening with very little effort, thereby providing more incentive for the patient to dress herself. Cotton leotards can be used as a substitute for both underwear and hose, in cold weather, for many patients. The leotards are available in many colors; the brighter colors are especially enjoyed by patients.

Shoes should be kept clean and in good repair. A type of shoe or sandal which does not require laces are most helpful when training patients to wear shoes. Sox and hose, or anklets, should be clean and free of holes. The use of stretch sox and hose makes it possible for every patient to have the correct size and fit. The use of panty-hose enables the female patient to appear better groomed, without wrinkled or falling hose.

There is no set time to start to teach a child to dress himself and there is no single way to train a child to dress himself. A few helpful ideas which have been learned from occupational therapists may be helpful:

1. First teach undressing, then go into the "how" of dressing and the handling of buttons and other fasteners.

2. Watch for signs that the child is ready to dress himself, such as the extending of an arm toward the garment.

3. Caution should always be taken to safeguard the child from falling. Many times their sense of balance is poor and a sturdy chair will provide the necessary support. If the sitting balance is poor, let the child put on some garments while he is still on the bed, as a pillow or the head of the bed forms a prop for part of the dressing procedure. If a child wants to try to put on any of his garments while in a wheelchair, be sure that the brakes are in the locked position.

4. Practice, with the child, the act of dressing, such as putting his hands and feet through the various motions of putting on a specific garment.

5. Practice with one garment at a time. Too many things are confusing.

6. Every procedure must be repeated not only once, but day after day, in some instances for months.
7. Directions must always be clear and concise, always the same. This is an excellent time to communicate as well as to instruct.
8. Help if necessary but do not be too obvious with your assistance. Start by placing the garments in order where the child can easily reach them.
9. Do not correct every little mistake. Making mistakes is one way of learning. Many times you will need to restrain yourself instead of taking over!
10. Learning the motor skills necessary in dressing oneself is one of the first steps toward greater skills, and coordination will develop through repetition.

It requires constant repetition and much patience on the part of the psychiatric technician who is training retarded patients to keep their clothes on and to present a neat, tidy appearance.

BEAUTY AND BARBER SHOP

Such facilities, under the supervision of trained operators, are usually available in the hospital for the use of ambulatory patients.

The hair of both boys and girls should be well brushed and combed. In so far as is possible patients should be taught to do this minimum amount of care. Neatness is facilitated by the use of short haircuts for boys and men. (A style known as the "butch-cut" is very practical.) Girls and women look more attractive if the hair cuts are not too short. Long hair presents a real nursing care problem unless the patient is capable of caring for it herself. Many mildly retarded females can learn how to care for their hair following a permanent. The familiar "home permanent" kits can be used on a ward, some patients being capable of learning how to fix their own hair.

The shape of the patient's head should always be taken into consideration when the hair is being dressed. The shaving of a patients head should not be done unless there is a doctor's order to do so. All patients should have a weekly shampoo.

For the adult male a daily shave is desirable whenever possible.

A minimum should be three times per week. The shaving procedure used will depend upon the hospital.

For the severely retarded and physically handicapped patients, the Psychiatric Technician must do the shampooing, the haircutting, the shaving and other personal grooming for the patients. Every patient should be given the opportunity to use a mirror and to learn what he looks like!

Teen age girls and adult females can be taught how to care for the skin of their hands and face, and how to use nail polish, lipstick, face powder and other make-up "secrets" to make themselves neat and attractive.

COMMUNICABLE DISEASES, THE PSYCHIATRIC TECHNICIAN AND THE PATIENT

Communicable diseases are also known as contagious or "catching" and many are known as "childhood diseases." Do not let the term "childhood diseases" mislead you because even though you may be an adult, you can catch them if you have not had them as a child.

Mentally retarded patients seem to be especially prone to catching any disease which is spread by discharges from the nose and throat. It would follow, therefore, that nursing personnel caring for the patients would also be likely to contract the disease too, if they had not had the disease.

An adult having one of these diseases is apt to be much sicker than a child. If a female employee becomes pregnant and is exposed to German measles and has the disease during the first three months of her pregnancy, it could have very serious effects on her unborn child. Abiding by common sense rules of good health will help you resist diseases: get enough sleep and rest, regular exercise and eat a well-balanced diet. It is also adviseable to have your vaccination against smallpox, as well as "shots" or immunization against polio, whooping cough, diphtheria and tetanus.

Being "immune" to a disease means that you can resist the infection. There are two types of immunity, *natural* and *acquired*. An acquired immunity is obtained by either having the disease by vaccination (against smallpox) or inoculations, such as are d(

for protection against diphtheria, whooping cough, scarlet fever, polio, typhoid fever and tetanus.

The diagnosis of any disease is made by the doctor. It is usually the psychiatric technician caring for the patients who will first notice the symptoms of illnesses, so prompt and accurate reporting of symptoms may prevent an epidemic from developing among the hospital population.

Common diseases which are spread by contact with a person having it and in which the discharges from the nose and throat are infectious are: chickenpox (varicella), diphtheria, German measles (rubella), measles (rubeola), mumps (infectious parotitis), whooping cough (pertussis), smallpox (variola), poliomyelitis (polio or infantile paralysis), and streptococcal sore throat (strep throat) including scarlet fever.

OBSERVATION OF PATIENTS

Early symptoms which the psychiatric technician can note and report to the doctor:

1. *Chicken pox*: First symptom in children is usually a rash often consisting of small blisters which have developed from small pimples.

2. *German measles*: May begin with mild symptoms of a cold in the head. Often times a rash is the first sign with a slight fever.

3. *Measles*: Begins with a fever, followed by symptoms like a cold in the head, running nose, sneezing and inflamed, watery eyes.

4. *Mumps*: Usually comes on suddenly with a fever and a swelling of the glands which are located at angle of the jaws.

5. *Whooping cough*: Symptoms may be mild at first, beginning with a cough which is worse at night.

6. *Poliomyelitis*: (Infantile paralysis)—sudden onset with fever, dull pain on bending neck forward, pain on being handled, headache and vomiting.

7. *Streptococcal sore throat*: Usually comes on suddenly with headache, fever, sore throat and often vomiting. If it is *scarlet fever* a fine, evenly distributed, red dot-like rash

appears within twenty-four hours, first on the neck and upper chest.

8. *Diphtheria*: In patients over one year of age the first symptom is usually a sore throat; in very young children the symptoms are like croup.

9. *Smallpox*: Usually comes on suddenly with a fever and severe backache; red pimples felt beneath the skin will appear on the exposed surfaces of the face and wrists about the third day.

POINTS TO REMEMBER WHEN CARING FOR PATIENTS WITH COMMUNICABLE DISEASES

1. The overall routine used is known as *isolation technique*. The specific procedures used will depend upon the hospital, the physical facilities available, and the doctor.

2. The technique is carried out to prevent the disease from spreading, to protect the patient from other infections and to protect the personnel caring for the patient.

3. *Things you can do*:
    a. Protect your clothing, or uniform, with a covering gown or apron.
    b. Wash your hands thoroughly after any contact with the patient.
    c. Keep your hands away from your face and mouth when caring for the patient and until you can wash your hands.
    d. Teach the patient to cover his nose and mouth with a handkerchief or paper tissue and turn his head away when sneezing or coughing.
    e. Do not give children toys that cannot be disinfected.

OTHER CONDITIONS WHICH CAN BE SERIOUS

1. The "*common cold*," although not usually listed as an official communicable disease, is very contagious. It occurs very frequently among mentally retarded patients. Those who have the ability should be trained how to use a hand-

kerchief or paper tissue when coughing or sneezing, how to blow their nose and keep it clean and to dispose of the used tissue or how to care for the handkerchief. A cold without complications is over within a few days. See that the patient has plenty of fluids to drink and keep at rest as much as is possible.

2. *Scabies*, or the itch, is spread by direct contact with the skin or clothing of a person who has it. It is more prone to occur where there is over-crowding plus poor personal hygiene. Absolute cleanliness of body, clothing and bed linens is the best method of prevention.

3. *Impetigo* is a fairly common condition which occurs among children and will spread rapidly unless treated immediately. It is prone to occur in epidemics in nurseries and children's wards in an institution. It begins as blisters, most often on the face and hands, and may be spread to other parts of the body by the child scratching with his fingernails. Good personal hygiene, plus frequent, thorough bathing is the best method of preventing this condition.

4. *Pinworms* frequently occur among groups of school-age children. The first symptom you may notice is the patient scratching around his anus, or bowel opening, especially at night. This is because itching is caused by the movement of the worms out of the bowel opening. This condition spreads rapidly through hand to mouth contact unless *strict* hygienic measures are taken: thorough washing of hands after toileting and before eating, frequent complete bathing with clean clothing from the skin out and change of bed linens.

   Medical treatment is prescribed by the doctor, an entire group or ward of patients usually being treated at the same time.

5. *Enteric* or intestinal diseases of certain types, occur frequently among mentally retarded patients. One of the most common is a dysentery which is caused by the parasite Entomoeba histolytica. Medical treatment is prescribed by the doctor. Nursing care emphasizes strict attention to cleanliness and good personal hygiene.

GIVING MEDICINE

The amount of responsibility given the psychiatric technician in regards to giving patients medications will depend upon the institution in which you work. If you are given this responsibility, it will usually be after you have had specific instructions about drugs, their effects and their dosages. You never give a medicine to a patient without a doctor's order, and if there is anything about the order which you do not understand, do not be afraid to ask for an explanation. It is much better for you to admit not knowing, if you are in doubt, than to endanger a patient's life by giving an incorrect medication.

RULES TO KEEP IN MIND WHEN GIVING MEDICINES

1. Have the order for the medicine signed by a doctor.
2. Know how to give the drug as prescribed.
3. Check carefully as to whether the dosage ordered is the same as that on the label. Although the doctor orders the dose, if you are giving the medicine you should have an idea of the difference between an adult dose and a child's dose. A commonly used rule for calculating a child's dose is *Young's Rule* $\dfrac{\text{Age}}{\text{Age} + 12} \times \text{adult dose} = \text{child's dose}.$
4. Prepare the medicine you give.
5. Have a good light when preparing medicines so that you read and see what you are doing.
6. Concentrate; let nothing distract your attention.
7. Read the label three times when preparing a medicine:
   a. When removing it from the shelf or drawer.
   b. After pouring or preparing it.
   c. When returning it to the shelf or drawer.
8. *Know your patient;* do not depend upon the patient for self identification nor upon a patient to identify another patient.
9. Stay with the patient until he *swallows* the medicine.
   a. Inspect the patient's mouth, asking him to open his

POURING MEDICINE

1. Hold label side up —
to keep label legible.

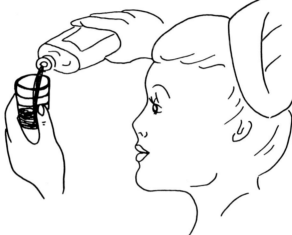

2. Medicine glass at eye level.

3. Thumbnail on mark.

MAINTAIN IDENTIFICATION
WITH MEDICINE CARD

Figure 24.

mouth, if there is any doubt in your mind that the medicine has not been swallowed. Some patients are very clever at concealing medications under the tongue or inside the cheek, for later disposal.

10. If a patient has difficulty in taking pills or capsules, sometimes the medicine can be dissolved in a liquid, or put into a spoonful of jelly or jam, to make it go down easier.

SYSTEMS OF WEIGHTS AND MEASURES

There are two systems in common use in measuring medicines, the "apothecary" and the "metric." The units of measure used in the apothecary system are of unequal size in relation to one another, where as the metric system is a decimal system with the units all bearing a relationship to each other based on ten or multiples of ten. There are also the common "household" measures which are sometimes used. A table showing the relationship between the three may be helpful to you:

Household Measure		*Apothecary Measure*		*Metric Measure*
Teaspoon	=	1 dram	=	4 c.c. (cubic centimeter)
Dessert spoon	=	2 drams	=	8 c.c.
Tablespoon	=	4 drams	=	15 c.c.
Cup	=	7 ounces	=	200 c.c.
Tumbler or glass	=	8 ounces	=	250 c.c.
Fruit jar	=	1 pint	=	500 c.c.
Fruit jar	=	1 quart	=	1000 c.c.

A table of weights used.

1 grain	=	0.065 Gm.
5 grains	=	0.3 Gm.
10 grains	=	0.6 Gm.
15 grains	=	1.0 Gm.

RESTRAINTS AND SECLUSION

The trend for many years has been to completely eliminate the use of restraining devices of any kind in the care and treatment of patients. Modern day useage of restraint varies from state to state and most psychiatrically oriented hospitals have definite rules and regulations governing the use of restraint. As a psychiatric technician you must know and understand the meaning of these rules.

The use of the "tranquilizer" drugs has greatly reduced the use of mechanical restraints, but there are times that a "tranquilizer" will not meet the patient's needs. A mechanical restraint is any device which interferes with the free movement of the patient and which he cannot remove. They may be classified as:

Medical: Used temporarily during an acute treatment such as the giving of a medicine by vein.

Supportive: Used to prevent helpless patients from falling out of chairs or beds, or as an assistance to patients while they are being fed, bathed or receiving other routine nursing care.

Behavioral: Used to prevent the patient from injuring himself or others, after other treatment measures have failed to control the patient's behavior.

Seclusion: The placing of a patient in a locked room by himself to prevent him from injuring himself or others.

Never use as punishment.

PRECAUTIONS TO OBSERVE

1. Use restraint only upon the order of the doctor.
2. Explain to the patient, if possible, why he is being restrained.
3. Do not make restraint too tight.

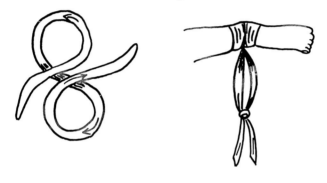

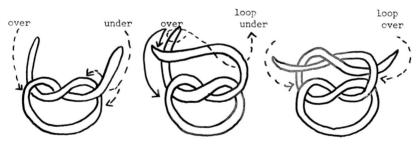

Figure 25. Soft cloth strips can be used to restrain hands. Twist the strip in the form of a figure 8 with the ends on top and extending in opposite directions. as shown in figure. The loops are put together and passed over the hand, a pad of soft material is inserted under them around the wrists and the ends of the strip drawn until the loops are small enough to prevent the hand being drawn through, but not tight enough to interfere with the circulation, the two ends are knotted together near the wrist and tied to the side of the bed or arm of the chair (as the case may be).

4. Do not apply restraint across the chest unless absolutely necessary.
5. Do not restrain only one side of the body; instead, restrain the right hand and the left foot, or vice versa.
6. Do not apply restraint in any way that will cause the circulation of the blood to be stopped.
7. Any restraining device should be in full view at all times, not covered by sheets and blankets, so that adequate observation can be made of the portions of the body which are restrained.
8. Protect the restrained patient from harm by other patients.
9. Never permit a patient to restrain another patient.
10. The chair in which a patient is restrained should be anchored to a non-moveable object, to prevent the chair from tipping over, and injuring the patient.

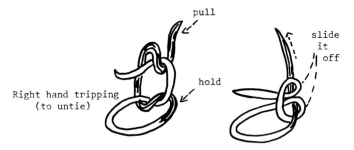

Figure 26. Square knot. The square knot should be used whenever it is necessary to tie any type of restraint, especially those made of cloth of any type. It holds securely, yet it can be easily untied. It is often tied incorrectly by crossing the ends improperly, it then becomes a granny knot which is insecure and also is liable to jam so that it cannot be untied.

PRINCIPLES OF NURSING CARE

1. Check the patient's pulse and general condition every 30 minutes, or more often.
2. Make the patient as comfortable as possible.
   a. Pad restraints to prevent bruising of skin.
   b. If in a room, have good ventilation.
   c. Do not fasten arms and/or legs in an exaggerated position.
3. Offer fluids at regular intervals. However, do not awaken for this reason if patient falls asleep.

4. Remove patient from restraint every two hours, take to the toilet, and give skin care such as an alcohol rub to the parts which have been restrained, before reapplying the restraint.

THINGS WHICH YOU CAN DO TO REDUCE THE NEED FOR BEHAVIORAL RESTRAINT

1. Know your patient's behavior patterns. An increased talkativeness, flushed face, restless pacing the floor, careless donning of clothing are just a few warning signs of approaching upset behavior. Occasionally a patient will have enough insight, or understanding, of his behavior that he will ask to be put in a room away from the other patients.

2. Give the patient something to do at which he can use his pent-up energy; such as: Calisthenics, games which can be played out-of-doors, ward work such as bedmaking, putting away linens, sweeping the floor, dusting; tearing rags for rug making, magazines for tearing (use magazines which have been read) and card games or checkers will sometimes interest the patient to the extent that he will slow down his activity in order to concentrate on the game.

3. Soft, nonstimulating music (no rock-n-roll) has a calming effect on some patients. (Use of a record player permits specific selection of music desired.)

4. A well-planned routine of occupational and recreational therapy can provide means for patients to work off excess energy as well as feelings of anger and hostility. A punching bag for instance, is much better for a patient to hit than for him to hit another patient.

5. Ideally, an excited, over-active, upset patient should have personalized attention from a psychiatric technician until he gets over his disturbed period. Unfortunately, too many hospitals do not have adequate staffing, so restraint or seclusion is substituted.

6. The use of hydrotherapy, in the form of cold wet sheet packs or continuous tub baths, is sometimes ordered for the treatment of over-active patients. The psychiatric technician does not perform these procedures unless they have been given spe-

cific instructions in their correct application by a licensed therapist, the doctor or a registered nurse.

SUGGESTIONS FOR HOLDING OR HANDLING RESISTIVE OR DISTURBED PATIENTS

There may be times when it is necessary to temporarily restrain and control a patient's movements. Examples of such instances are: the necessity for carrying out a nursing care procedure, the need for a physical examination of a specific area of the body, or disturbed behavior. You should then be aware of the following:

1. Type of restraint must not injure the patient.
2. At least two persons should carry out such restraints.
3. Plan your maneuvers in advance.
4. At the sign of approaching trouble remove your own glasses if you wear them, watch, fountain pen or anything of value.
5. If the patient is wearing shoes with "hard" soles, remove the shoes to prevent injury to others.
6. If a female patient is mildly excited, it may be sufficient to walk beside her, placing an arm around her waist and grasping the wrist of the forearm with your hand; with your other hand grasp the wrist of the patient's other arm drawn toward the front of the body. The other person should walk on the other side of the patient.
7. Do not touch a male patient, the employees should walk one on each side of the patient. If necessary, take hold of an arm, flex the arm at the elbow, and place your arm between the patient's arm and body and clasp the wrist. Walk with the patient, all walking forward. If the patient is hard to manage use the same method as above except that the patient's arms are drawn to the back. Have the patient walk backward, the nursing employees walk forward.
8. All workers should know where the patient is being taken, if he is being moved, so that they move in the same direction.
9. To prevent biting, scratching, and hitting, keep behind the patient or at the side; if you take hold of the patient's arm, grasp the wrist.
10. Never take hold of an excited patient by the hand and pull

forward; the patient immediately pulls backward and has control of his maximum strength.

11. In applying pressure, as in holding a wrist, have some cloth between the patient's flesh and your hand; this reduces the possibility of bruising. Hold on to the patient but exert pressure only when necessary. *Never* exert pressure over the chest.

12. If the patient has a dangerous object such as a hammer or knife, place first attention on the article. If necessary throw something—a sheet, a blanket or a large garment—over the patient's face. Use a mattress as a shield. In extreme situations approach the patient from behind.

ACCIDENTS DO HAPPEN

Just as accidents will occasionally occur in your home, so will they occasionally occur in the patient's home, the ward or cottage. The more people there are in a "home" and the more activities there are, the greater the likelihood will be that accidents may occur. While it should not be considered a disgrace to have an incident on your ward, you, the psychiatric technician should make every effort to eliminate any situation which would permit a recurrence of the same incident. Prevention is always better than the cure! You must be alert at all times to protect the patient from self injury or from inflicting injury on others.

In an institutional setting where a doctor is on call at all times, the amount of first aid performed by psychiatric technicians is usually not extensive and is, as a rule, defined by specific rules and regulations. Many institutions give specific courses in First Aid using the American Red Cross First Aid Textbook for their instructions. Knowledge gained from such a course would enable you to know what to do, skillfully and quickly, before the doctor arrives. For instance, if a patient should cut an artery, the action you take may be a matter of life or death for that patient.

Incidents which frequently occur with children of all ages are: (1) bruises, cuts and lacerations of varying degree; (2) foreign objects in the ears or nose; (3) fractures and dislocations; (4) choking due to aspiration of food, vomitus or a foreign body; (5) swallowing a poisonous material; (6) over-exposure to the sun, and (7) burns.

Many other emergency situations can occur, such as drowning, bleeding from any part of the body, or over-exposure to the cold.

Call your supervisor as soon as possible when an incident occurs (some institutions will instruct you to call the doctor first).

BRUISES, CUTS, LACERATIONS

These may occur to some extent just in the process of living, working and playing together in large groups such as are found in any institutional setting. Scuffles and quarrelling among patients, activities involving toys, play equipment and tools, patients falling when having seizures and over-active patients breaking windows with their fists, are just a few of the occasions which produce incidents. Close observation and supervision of the patients at all times by the psychiatric technician can do much to prevent incidents occurring.

Any wound should be kept as clean as possible and bleeding should be stopped. If the bleeding is severe, you cannot wait for the doctor to take action. You must stop the bleeding by applying pressure directly against the bleeding point, preferably by placing the cleanest material at hand over the spot, then pressing against the spot with your hand. You may have to use your bare hand in order to save the patient's life.

Sometimes when a patient is badly hurt, he will go into a state of shock. Signs of shock which you can recognize are:

1. The skin is pale, cold, and moist feeling.
2. The breathing is shallow and irregular.
3. The pulse is weak and rapid.
4. The pupils of the eyes are usually dilated.

Keep the patient quiet and cover with a blanket or other covering until assistance arrives.

FOREIGN OBJECTS IN EARS AND NOSE

Buttons, pieces of toys, beans, pieces of food, bugs and any one of a multitude of objects that can be picked up by a patient, on a ward or out-of-doors, may be pushed into an ear or up the nose.

The technician should not try to remove the object but call the supervisor and/or the doctor.

FRACTURES AND DISLOCATIONS

Bones may be broken or dislocated for many reasons: Too rough play activities among young and energetic patients; slips and falls

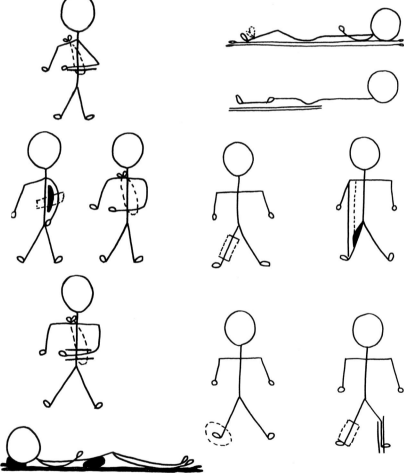

Figure 27. Diagrams on Fracture First Aid

1. Fracture of Arm—One splint, cravat arm sling, cravat to bind arm to chest.
2. Elbow—(a) If found bent arm sling only; bind arm to body. (b) If found straight one splint, arm may be bound to side of body; pad armpit very well.

among older patients because of too highly waxed floors, or wet spots on the floor, or poorly placed scatter rugs. Infirm patients may fall out of bed due to improperly fastened siderails. Technicians can do much to prevent such incidents by being alert and aware of what the patients under their supervision are doing at all times. Good ward housekeeping will eliminate many safety hazards. Patients who are unsteady on their feet should be assisted in getting about. The use of an invalid walker does much to make them feel less dependent.

If an accident does occur, you should not move the patient unless absolutely necessary. However, if the accident occurs when a patient is engaged in an off-ward activity, such as on a hike, a picnic or on a work assignment, he will have to be moved. Any sprain, strain or suspected dislocation or fracture should be treated as a fracture, the patient being kept quiet until assistance arrives, and a splint being applied before any moving occurs.

CHOKING

Choking on food is one of the most common causes of suffocation, or stoppage of breathing. This may occur at meal time if a patient eats too rapidly, or if a patient grabs food and crams it into his mouth and down his throat. Quick action is necessary on the part of the psychiatric technician, to remove this obstruction to the patient's breathing. A quick blow with the palm of the hand on the patient's back between the shoulder blades, may dislodge the ob-

---

3. Forearm and Wrist—Two splints, arm sling.
4. Spine—Small pad in small of back; transport on firm frame, on back; support head, especially if fracture is high.
5. Pelvis—Transport on firm frame, on back. Bind knees and ankles together. Flex knees if more comfortable.
6. Knee Cap—One splint, buttocks to heel, behind extremity.
7. Thigh—One splint, armpit to foot. Second splint, shoulder to heel behind extremity may be applied.
8. Leg—Pillow or blanket, perhaps with two wood splints outside, or two splints alone.
9. Ankle—Pillow or blanket about leg and ankle or two splints, heel to knee.
10. Foot Fracture or Crushing—Large, loose padded dressing or pillow or blanket.

ject. Otherwise, the object may be removed with your fingers if precautions are taken to prevent the patient from biting your fingers.

A bed patient may aspirate, or breathe into the lungs, particles of food or liquid when being fed. He will start gasping, his lips turn blueish color and he may stop breathing. Call for help but do not leave the patient. Start artificial respiration and continue until assistance arrives.

Any patient, especially those who are bedfast, are in potential danger if they vomit. Unless they are given prompt attention they actually choke to death on the vomited material, as they start gasping and struggling for air, in the process drawing the foreign material into the lungs.

SWALLOWING POISONOUS MATERIALS

Fly and insect sprays, cleaning agents of many varieties and medications of any kind may be accidentally, or intentionally, swallowed by patients. Whenever this occurs it is usually due to an employee's carelessness in leaving such materials unsupervised, or leaving a medicine cupboard unlocked, or leaving doors to treatment or supply rooms unlocked.

If the technician thinks a patient has swallowed anything of a poisonous nature, call the supervisor and/or the doctor immediately. Do not give an antidote, or remedy to counteract the poison, unless you are *sure* that it will produce the desired effect.

OVER-EXPOSURE TO THE SUN

This can be prevented by the patients being properly dressed for outside activities during hot weather. Patients should wear hats for example, if they are going out in mid-day in the Summer time. The amount of activity at any one time should be restricted on a hot day. If working outside, rest periods should be taken in the shade.

If a patient is overcome by the heat of the sun, keep him quiet and shaded and call the doctor.

BURNS

Burns may be caused by dry or moist heat.

Patients who smoke may accidentally burn themselves, or set fire to their clothing, or set fire to bedding or other objects unless properly supervised. Patients who have seizures may fall against heat sources such as steam radiators or electrical devices. Patients sometimes tamper with electrical outlets and in addition to being burned, receive a severe shock.

Patients may be accidentally burned when being bathed, or unsupervised patients may turn on hot water and scald themselves or other patients.

Ward decorations as for a special occasion, such as Christmas season, should always be fire proofed.

If a patient's clothing is on fire, smother the flames, and remove clothing. Do not attempt to remove anything burned into the flesh. Call the doctor and supervisor. Do not use anything to treat the patient until the doctor gives an order. (Much harm can be done by the improper use of ointments, salves and similar substances.)

DROWNING

All patients must be closely supervised at any time they have access to swimming pools, or are near or in water (such as on bath day), to prevent accidental drowning. Bathroom doors should be kept locked when the bathroom is not being used.

If such an accident does occur, get the patient out of the water, turn him on his stomach, turn his face to one side and check that the tongue has not fallen back in the throat. Start artificial respiration and continue until assistance arrives. Call for the supervisor.

DIVERSIONAL ACTIVITIES FOR PATIENTS

There are many therapists who have specialties: occupational, recreational, music, just to name a few. Anyone who has contact with the patients shares, to some extent, the responsibility for patient activity. The psychiatric technician carries the greatest responsibility for activities on the ward; however, because they are the personnel who are always with the patients. You are the ones who must initiate a ward program. It will depend upon the hospital as to what facilities are available and as to how many therapists there are to call upon for assistance.

Activities will not do the impossible. There is no magic word or game that will suddenly quiet your hyperactive patients or make your quiet patients jump up and play. The most important single thing that will determine the success or failure of an activities program on your ward is your attitude. You will have to be genuinely interested not only in the patient, but in the game or activity which you are trying to put across. Be alert to each patient, find out who the shy ones are and who are the leaders. Consult with the therapist as to ideas for activities and games and for help as to how to handle a certain group.

APPROACHES YOU CAN USE IN PRESENTING ACTIVITIES

1. *Repetition.* Don't expect the child to understand the first time through; repeat and repeat.
2. *Imitation.* Don't tell him how to do or play something; *show* him.
3. *Praise.* Be sure to praise the child for something he has done well according to his ability.
   The ideal program would be one which would fit the child, *not* fit the child into the program.

METHODS OF CONTROL THAT YOU MIGHT TRY IF CERTAIN PATIENTS ARE DISRUPTING THE ACTIVITY

1. Speaking repeatedly to the patient.
2. Redirecting his interest to something else.
3. Isolating the patient from the rest of the group.
4. Depriving the patient of the activity.

You Will Have Success With the Activities You Lead If You

1. *Split your group*: Try a small group of patients first. The others will join in the activity as they become interested.

2. *Know how to play the game* yourself before attempting to teach it to others.

3. *Get the attention of the group*: Speak where everyone in the group can see you; speak to be heard but do not shout.

4. *Demonstrate the activity*; make sure that all understand how to play.

5. *Play in the game yourself*: Interest in the activity will lag if you just give directions and then stand aside.

6. *Keep things moving*: Use variations of the game being played.

7. *Stop the activity* at peak of interest, not after everyone is tired of it.

8. *Vary the games played* and alternate the activities as to quiet and energetic.

9. *Learn to adapt activities* to the patient's level of ability. An *active* circle game can be converted to a quiet game by having the patients *sit* in a circle. A teen-ager may not want to play a "baby" game even though that may be all that they are mentally capable of understanding!

10. *Try to teach games that the patients can* play by themselves when you are not present.

11. *Use recognized leaders* within the patient group. There are always ring-leaders on a ward that the group as a whole will follow; use these leaders as "helpers."

12. *Recognize that the mentally retarded* patients are different in their play and adapt accordingly. For example, if everyone in the group wants to be "It", let them and choose someone to be "Not it." The use of music as therapy can be adapted to meet the needs of vastly different types of patients and any size of group. It can be used for all ages and mentalities. It can ease tensions and it can stimulate the listless. By the use of a record player and a record of some simple folk dance music, quite retarded ambulatory patients can be stimulated to basic activity such as joining hands in a circle and walking around. Playing, singing, talking, laughing, listening; any activity done with a patient can be therapeutic. For example of specific activities and directions for doing them, see appendix A.

ACTIVITIES FOR BEDFAST PATIENTS

There are more things to do for this group than you might at first think possible. The majority can see and hear, but for those who can neither see nor hear as well as being bedfast, the scope of activities *is* limited. A little extra personalized attention when feeding them, and when bathing and giving bedside care, can always be done.

Music: Many variations are possible, such as radio, or a record player, or singing, such as you would do when caring for any child.

Pictures: Many patients enjoy bright, colorful pictures. Ward decorations give you an opportunity to use your imagination in providing a relief from monotony for bed patients. Decorate to fit the season or special occasion, such as Valentine Day, Easter or Christmas. Color books and picture magazines are enjoyed by some. Television, when available, is enjoyed by many bedfast patients. The movement of the picture as well as the sound provides diversion. Colorful mobiles, suspended from the ceiling or any archway, provide entertainment for children.

Toys: The majority of patients (mentally retarded adult and child) enjoy toys. Toys should be washable, colorful, soft and cuddly, and not too big. Toys which can be attached to cribs are enjoyed by patients.

Out-door Activities: These are in most instances restricted. Sometimes the cribs or beds can be rolled out of the ward, into a yard area, and the patients get a sunbath. For a special treat, they can be given a "picnic" instead of their regular lunch, the food being modified for the occasion, and eaten out-of-doors, the beds being taken out into the yard.

Patients can also be put on a blanket or pad, spread in the yard, to provide an opportunity for them to be outside.

Sometimes even the most severely handicapped patients can be taken for a "walk" or "ride." This is dependent upon sufficient personnel to prepare the patients and wheelchairs or other wheeled equipment. (A child's little red wagon is suitable for a small patient.)

VOCATIONAL TRAINING

Introduction

Mentally retarded individuals with an intellectual potential ranging from the moderately retarded to the borderline level are employable, if they have had adequate training. This training must start early, even earlier than is done with normal children, with much repetition and endless patience on the part of the teacher being required. Emphasis during the training years is on social adjustment; i.e., to develop habits and attitudes that will make it easier for the patient to get a job and to be able to hold the job after he does get it.

The academic school of any institution for the mentally retarded usually gives the formal instruction in the 3 R's: reading, 'riting and 'rithmetic, as any patient must acquire a minimum knowledge in these subjects if he is to live outside of the protective environment of an institution. For example, reading is necessary to be able to understand street signs, price labels and warning signs such as *Stop*; knowledge of arithmetic to the extent that he can make change, pay for articles he may purchase and be able to know whether he receives the correct change, and know enough about writing to sign his name to fill in forms. He should also be able to tell time.

WHAT THE PSYCHIATRIC TECHNICIAN DOES

It is at the ward level that desirable attitudes and socially acceptable behavior is stressed and encouraged, the earlier in the patient's life the better. The attitude and interest of the psychiatric technician cannot be over emphasized. Just as a father and mother would do with their own child, the technicians must teach the patients to care for their personal appearance, to speak so that they can be understood, to have good manners, to get along with others, to follow orders when given, to complete a job once begun and to master the multitude of lessons which must be learned if the patient is to adjust to society.

The psychiatric technician should never underestimate the ability of a patient; in fact, he should be eager to encourage the patients to try new activities, at the same time emphasizing the importance of completing one task before starting another. Any assignment should be within the range of the patient's ability to perform and they will need to be *shown* how to do the job, rather than just be *told*. The majority of ambulatory patients, both male and female, can learn how to make their own bed and to do other types of "housework" such as sweeping, mopping, dusting, window washing and other tasks to help keep their home ward neat and clean. Many can learn to care for their own clothing and shoes and to pick up after themselves.

The psychiatric technician should work closely with the occupational therapists and the industrial therapist in developing activity programs which can best develop the potential ability of every patient.

OCCUPATIONAL THERAPY

In a way, occupational therapy can be thought of as pre-vocational training for retarded patients. It should be more than just "busy" work; rather, a real project of which he can feel proud when it is completed. The activities should consist of a variety of experiences not just the crafts. The opportunity to become acquainted with various tools, materials and equipment can be provided through gardening, wood-working, painting or clay modeling, to name a few. Modeling clay because of its softness is easier for a patient to use who is learning how to use both hands at once, than a solid object. Many occupational therapy projects can be initiated at ward level by the psychiatric technician for the patients.

A few examples would be leathercrafts, sewing, rugmaking and certain types of woodcraft. A specific example of a completed project: A group of adolescent, moderately to mildly retarded boys constructed fences for the flower beds outside their ward. Under the close supervision of a psychiatric technician, the boys used an electric saw to cut discarded broom handles into the desired lengths, put them together and painted them a bright yellow. The patients were given a feeling of pride and achievement in that they had improved the appearance of their "home"!

As a rule, the patient's attention span is relatively short, so much repetition and encouragement is required. Eventually, the patient will be capable of being "promoted" to an industrial therapy assignment.

INDUSTRIAL THERAPY

Assignments in industrial therapy should be provided to give the patient an opportunity to work under different conditions and under different supervisors. Future employers are not so much concerned with whether the mentally retarded applicant can perform technical skills, but rather, is he habit trained, is he honest, can he be relied upon to do his job and will he be able to get along with his fellow workers as well as with the boss. Much can be done by the therapists and the psychiatric technician in teaching patients these habits.

Industrial therapy is usually thought of as placement of patients in occupational situations within an institution, and should be based upon the needs of the patient. In some states the responsibility for this type of vocational training rests with the Department of Education and the institutional industries are used as training programs.

There are no short-cuts to learning, or "summer jobs" available for the mentally retarded. Like anyone else, they will do a job well if it is within their range of competence and they feel comfortable and happy in doing it. As with every educational and training pro-

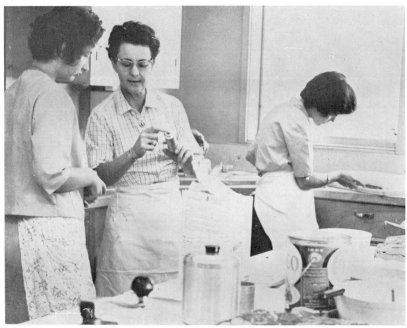

Figure 28. Vocational training. Adolescent girls learning how to bake and decorate cakes. Courtesy: Porterville State Hospital, Porterville, California.

gram for the retarded individual, vocational training requires constant, consistent supervision in repetitive jobs. The employees responsible for the patients' training, as well as any future employee, must have a positive attitude and the patience to repeat demonstrations as long as necessary to obtain the correct performance of the task being taught. Once a mentally retarded individual has learned a routine he does it well and he sticks to it, performing it in the same way over and over again. For those who do progress to employment,

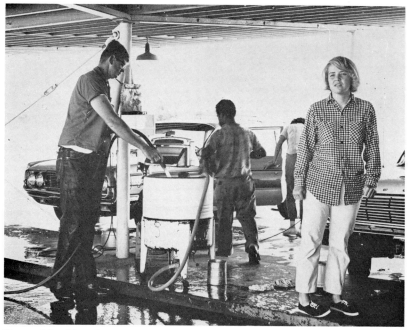

Figure 29. Vocational training. Adolescent boys and girls learning correct work methods while washing cars. Courtesy: Porterville State Hospital, Porterville, California.

it will be for most a job in the unskilled or semi-skilled categories such as attending machines, performing simple hand operations, filling station attendant, messengers or farmhands. The availability of employment will depend upon the community, whether it be a rural area or an urban one. (See appendix B for specific jobs possible for different age levels.)

The principles related to the supervision of the retarded "Vocational Trainee," whether it is the vocational training employee, or the employer in the community, are the same.

Remember that,

1. They think more slowly.
2. It takes more time and patience to get them started.
3. They get confused and may not be able to act, if you give them too many instructions at once or if the instruction is too complicated.

When supervising:

1. Tell him things clearly, directly and simply.
2. Show, whenever possible, how the task is to be done.
3. Correct his mistakes.
4. Give credit for a job well done. A pat on the back is good for anyone.
5. Encourage him to do his job; let him feel that he is in a job that is not constantly changing.

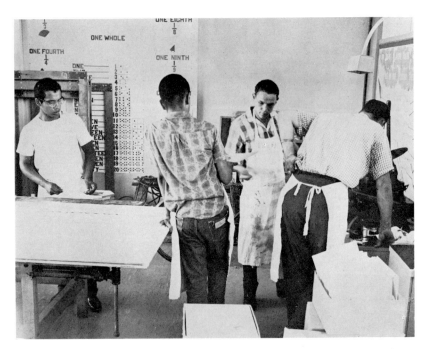

Figure 30. Vocational training. Boys learning how to make correct calculations in shop work. Courtesy: Porterville State Hospital, Porterville, California.

6. Don't feel that you must watch him constantly; taper off your supervision as he shows that he can handle the job.

7. Don't use complicated language or give half-explanations; make your directions specific, clear, concrete and complete. Give your instructions slowly and one step at a time.

8. Treat him as an adult even though he is less able than others in the thinking and learning process.

9. Don't be too busy or uninterested to make sure that all is going well. Be available for counselling or to provide a listening ear.

10. And last but not least, don't feel sorry for him.

There is much yet to be done in the training and preparation of the mentally retarded for their place in society as first class citizens. There is no reason why a retardate who has been well trained cannot be employed, as "stability" is a good word to sum up many of his attributes. They will also stick with routine without getting restless, they try hard to please and will take pride in their work. An employer will have no trouble if he remembers to do the same thing as with any other employee, only a little less at a time, a bit more slowly, and to use very simple words when doing his instructing.

RELIGIOUS TRAINING

General

Hospitals, state schools and other institutions will usually have chaplains on their staffs representing the three major faiths, the Protestant, the Catholic and the Jewish.

Both the psychiatric technician and the registered nurse should have an awareness and understanding of the practices and holy days associated with each faith. This knowledge facilitates both the instruction of the patients and the assistance given those patients who are capable of participating in the appropriate activity.

The Protestant faith embraces a large number of denominations. Each has practices and interpretations uniquely its own.

There are many ceremonies related to the practice of the Catholic faith which are very important to a patient. For those who are capable of partaking, Confession and Holy Communion are usually scheduled at designated intervals. A combination of sacraments, commonly referred to as the "last rites," are administered to a Catholic patient who is in danger of dying. Last rites are very important to a Catholic patient and it is imperative that the technician or nurse notify the priest in time to administer them, no matter at what hour of the day or night the patient's condition seems to warrant it.

The Sabbath day for those of the Jewish faith extends from after sunset on Friday until after sunset on Saturday. There are many dietary regulations related to the Jewish religion, i.e., kosher or sanctioned by Jewish law, especially designating food that may be eaten as ritually clean. However, Jewish law permits a patient to eat whatever the physician prescribes for his health. Passover and the eight-day period following is observed annually by those of the Jewish faith. Should a Jewish patient die who has no known relatives, a rabbi should be contacted.

Training

Parents are always concerned as to whether their children will be able to take part in religious services and are happy to learn that this can be.

Every child has the right to a Christian education and even the severely retarded can benefit from special classes which are keyed to their mental abilities. Much more simplified instruction

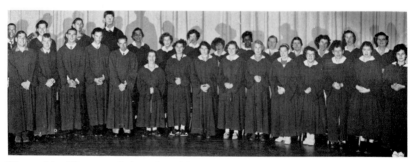

Figure 31. The retarded patients' love of music and rhythm resulted in this group of boys and girls learning, by constant repetition, many hymns as well as other types of songs. The program, originated as part of the patients' religious education, resulted in valuable community contacts, as they have given many performances for community groups. The musical direction was provided by a volunteer. Courtesy of Porterville State Hospital, Porterville, California.

and repetition as well as more visual aids are needed in teaching these children. Many can learn to repeat a simple "grace" when seated at the table, before eating their meal. The technician can teach them this basic lesson even though the patients may not attend formal church services.

Retarded children love music and it has been observed that in Sunday school sessions, they can learn a great deal from songs, especially if the words refer to things they know and understand.

For the patients whose vocational training has reached the point where he can return to the community, a knowledge of church services can be of great comfort to him. The need for social activities are all too often denied the retarded person and in many instances a church group can aid in filling the gap.

No matter how much the technician or the doctor can offer reassurance to the parents of a retarded child, it is not the comfort that the hospital chaplain can offer them. The chaplain helps many parents to overcome their feelings of guilt because they have placed their child in an institution and reassures them of God's love and grace.

ROLE OF THE VOLUNTEER

The use of volunteers in mental hospitals is not new. As far back as World War I the Grey Ladies worked on hospital treatment wards as volunteers.

In the advancement of treatment processes for the mentally ill and the mentally retarded there has been established a service which has greater importance than was ever attributed to it in its developmental stage; that is, the use of volunteers as a supplement to the technical and professional staff of mental hospitals.

The treatment of patients involves the use of highly trained staffs and carefully planned hospitals, the aim of all treatment being to bring the mentally ill patient into contact once again with reality and society, and to prepare the mentally retarded for acceptance by society. State hospital staffs are of less than optimum size; indeed, it is the exception rather than the rule if a state institution has a nursing staff large enough to provide the maximum in therapeutic services to its patients. It is for this reason that the services of various volunteer groups are usually more than welcomed. With the help of volunteers the work of the hospital nursing staff can be extended tremendously. Volunteers come from many sources: A woman whose family has grown up and moved away, leaving her with time to spare; a young people's club or organization, a church group, or it may be a friend or relative of a patient in the hospital. These people offer their services with no desire for a monetary reward; their only wish (with only rare exceptions) being a sincere one of wanting to help those who are less fortunate than they.

The volunteer on the ward working with patients is constantly offering the patient contact with reality and in so doing is contributing to his progress toward recovery. Patients must have these contacts with the outside world, in order to learn and gain confidence enough to face life outside the hospital. These personal contacts come from the community by those in the community working within the hospital as volunteers and by the acceptance of patients into the community through attendance and participation in social functions, tours, athletic events, civic meetings, shopping trips, and many other occasions.

The psychiatric technician should make every effort to cooperate with and be of assistance to any volunteer worker when the latter is providing an activity of any kind for the patients on his ward.

The services of volunteer workers in a specific hospital are usually coordinated by some member of the hospital staff, perhaps in connection with the Rehabilitation Therapies Department.

Some hospitals have a "Friendship Service" for patients whose chief hope for personal friendship is from an individual or group sponsor outside the hospital. This work is done by volunteer workers with the information about the patient's wishes, needs, sizes in wearing apparel, as well as that about the patient's behavior being provided by the psychiatric technician. Sometimes this information is transmitted to the volunteer worker by the coordinator.

In addition to their work within the hospital, volunteers are invaluable interpreters of the newer concepts of treatment and of the function of the mental hospital in relationship to the community. They can aid in dispelling many of the false beliefs related to both mental illness and mental retardation. The basic role of the volunteer in a state hospital setting consists of several facets: (1) to act in a supplemental capacity to staff in helping patients, (2) to interpret to the community the new concepts of mental illness and mental retardation and progress being made in treatment methods, and (3) where it is appropriate to inform the community of the problems and needs of the hospital staff.

The volunteer can be thought of somewhat in terms of a bridge— the two ends of which are the volunteers within the hospital and the volunteers within the community. Volunteers can form a bridge of knowledge and support, from hospital to community, across which the mentally ill and the mentally retarded patient can return, with increasingly less hospitalization, to a normal life.

PSYCHOTHERAPY

Introduction

To the uninitiated, the word "psychotherapy," and related terms, has for many years presented a mysterious barrier which could not be passed unless one could verbalize freely and fluently in the "jargon."

Psychotherapy as it relates to that which is done by nursing personnel (registered nurses, psychiatric technicians, ward aides or attendants) need not be mysterious at all if it is borne in mind that it is basically the process of sharing an experience with a patient.

The mere fact that a session of any type; a small group, a large group, or an individual one-to-one type situation, is called a "therapy session" does not necessarily mean that therapy has occurred. Both the patient and the therapist must be considered in any such inter-action even though one does not always have the answer as to what does happen. However, some of the things that the therapist does that might be therapeutic are:

1. *He listens*, allowing the patient to talk implies some degree of acceptance which in turn gives the patient an idea of worth.
2. *He talks*, this gives the patient the feeling that he is worth talking to.
3. *He asks questions*, this gives the patient the feeling that the therapist is really concerned about his welfare.

4. *He acts in an accepting manner.*

5. *He socializes* the patient into a new role. The patient learns that self-control is expected.

GROUP THERAPY WITH THE MENTALLY RETARDED

Group therapy for the mentally retarded patient is the most valuable form of psychotherapy. The mentally retarded who have been in institutions for any period of time at all are deficient in terms of gratification of basic needs: love, attention, encouragement, praise, respect, as well as many other needs. Due to this deprivation they too fall heir to feelings of insecurity, anxiety, rejection and uncertainty. Any person who chooses to work with and care for the mentally retarded must always bear in mind that the retardate is quite sensitive and has a great capacity for warm, human relationships.

Ward nursing personnel, who spend the greatest number of hours with the patients, can carry out group therapy under proper training and supervision. Above all other qualifications, the therapist must have a humane and sympathetic feeling for the mentally retarded patient, coupled with the ability to create a warm, permissive atmosphere that is bounded by definite limits. In the role of therapist, the nursing person can have no reservations about respecting the patient, and accepting him as he truly is. The particular approach to be used can best be determined in terms of the needs of each individual patient. Chronological age presents no real barrier in relation to benefits which may be derived from group therapy. And in some instances, the employee will benefit as much, perhaps more so than the patients who participate in group therapy sessions.

What is done and what occurs in the course of group therapy can perhaps be best explained, in part, by quoting from combined reports which have been given by psychiatric technicians who have participated in a basic program pertaining to group therapy.

Report No. 1

My selected group was composed of six moderately retarded elderly women, ranging in age from 33 to 77 years. All are able to verbalize.

Objectives: How to recognize the value of group therapy, how to apply what I have learned in classes and to promote better feelings between patient 'R' and the other people on the ward.

First meeting revealed: 'Granny' is the dominant one and assumed the role of leader. 'M' took part in a mild, ineffectual way, 'E' was talkative but cooperative. 'T' spoke only when called on and midway of the meeting she turned her back on the group. 'G' contributed to the discussion but had little impression as it is difficult to understand her. Outside influence on the group was other patients looking through the window and the instructor's visit. Inside influence was my guiding of the conversation in the direction I wished it to go at times.

A later session: We fixed a pitcher of Koolaid to drink while we held our meeting seated around a table in the ward dining room. The discussion started with reminiscing about yesterday's swimming party. It seemed like more fun to them looking back on it than when it was actually taking place.

Later: . . . 'M' actually hates 'R.' None of them want her to touch them. . . . we have not achieved our goal of improving relationships with 'R,' they still dislike her but they have learned to conceal it to a certain extent . . . they have learned to converse with each other more freely.

Conclusions:

1. I should have selected a different goal and let improving relations be the hidden agenda. (This trying to improve relations with 'R' developed a 'righteous' attitude in some of the members.)
2. It would have been better to have selected a group from some ward other than my own.
   a. They were too anxious to please me.
   b. Other patients on the ward found it hard to understand why we did not take turns as we do in other things.
   c. I had preconceived ideas as to their ability. I found myself wrong sometimes and probably would have made more progress if I had expected more of them or had had an open mind.
3. I learned that to live in a large group for 24 hrs. a day, year after year, it is necessary to develop a strong protective shell. They are able to shut out people so well it is as though they

are not in the room at all. At first I was amazed to find that they all had this trait. In trying to understand it I began imagining myself as living with 70 or 80 people. No privacy and very few opportunities to be alone, and I came to the conclusion that the only way you could survive would be to be able to 'wall' yourself off. Learn to be alone in a crowd.

4. To hold the interest, a variety of activities should be planned.
5. There is less communication when a group is involved with physical activity.
6. Simple projects that can be completed successfully in a short period of time are best. Some of the things we used were:
   a. Play school wooden puzzle (about fifteen pieces).
   b. Play school wooden blocks of different shapes and color that may be used to form different designs.
   c. Common A B C blocks.
   d. Flannel picture making sets.
   e. Tea party.
   f. Picnic.
   g. Swimming party.
7. Older people do not like to be active and occupied all the time. They enjoy their resting, dozing and reminiscing.
8. I found that you can accomplish much if you listen more than you talk.

Report No. 2

Selection of the Group: Four boys, each of whom has need to be motivated to relate more warmly and more naturally with others living on their ward. They are moderately to mildly mentally retarded. *Ray,* twenty years of age, but small, is withdrawn, quiet and passive with spasticity of extremities appearing to always stand on the outer edge of large groups as though too timid to offer anything for fear of being unaccepted. *Frank,* twelve years old, is very verbal and has a terrific need to be needed. When he seems frustrated by the day's events he will occasionally resort to tearful outbursts and regressive behavior. At these times he is content to lay in bed in a near fetal position, refusing to eat unless coaxed into each bite of food and each swallow of liquid. *Jack,* ten years old, is anxious and passive but easily aggravated to disturbed behavior and is diagnosed as having epilepsy. He presents a nonverbal figure, has a pleasant smile and responsive attitude to simple instructions until he feels he cannot give the expected as well as some other child. At these times he is likely to throw objects about wildly, fall to the floor and completely disrobe himself. *Barry*, ten years old, is mischievous, charming and at times thoroughly distracting. He is almost always negativistic, even to the point of almost defeating his own aims. He does show the ability to assume more responsibility for his own actions. He has never related warmly to anyone, this being apparent even as an infant.

Chief Purpose and Goal

Acceptable activity and motivation for individual and independent action according to individual need and functional ability. Each patient will therefore, be happier and better able to conform to certain behavior standards which will enable him to have more freedom. A permissive approach will be used in solving

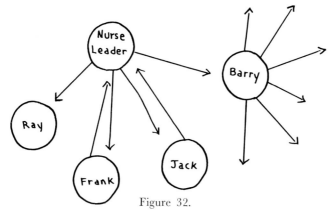

Figure 32.

this group's problems. Limitations will be based upon safety factors and feelings of security for the individuals.

First Meeting: Sociogram No. 1 indicates the degree of activity. *Frank* and *Jack* were eager but reflected dependency upon me which did not seem unusual to me since this was a completely new situation for all of them and they were not sure of their roles. *Barry* was unusually busy, all non-directed activity, completely independent of the others. *Ray* was very quiet but since he reflected no desire to leave I believe he was interested.

Sixth Session: The boys had a scheduled bus ride at 3:00 P.M. today. The bus rides mean a great deal to Ray, Frank and Jack, Barry is not usually allowed to go because of his disruptive be-

havior. So rather than interfere or have them feel they must decide between the bus ride or our meeting, I decided to take
Barry and we would all go on the ride as there was adequate
seating. I met with some resistance from the ward personnel because of their previous experience with Barry on bus rides. I
reminded them that these four boys were my responsibility and
not theirs on this particular ride; so they relaxed their anxieties
and settled down to watch the 'fun' and off on the bus we went.
For the first ten to fifteen minutes my small group appeared to
have become 'one-to-one' with Barry the other 'one.' After much
guilt talk and encouragement to look at the fun the other boys
were having and reminders that we would not be able to go on
any more rides if he (Barry) couldn't settle down, he finally
began to look out the window and soon pointed out certain
things and made efforts to establish verbal communications between himself and the other boys. Of course, he continued to
need reassurance from me that 'all was well' but all in all I
believe we made progress.

Seventh Session: Frank was ill today and unable to join us for
our hour of play therapy. 'Progress' sociogram No. 2 reflects
the attitude of the remaining three. Perhaps Frank's absence
was instrumental in Barry feeling that he must see after Ray. As

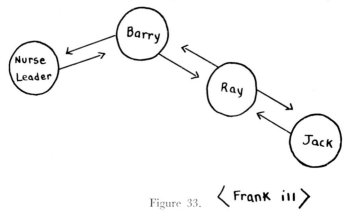

Figure 33.   ⟨ Frank ill ⟩

we went on a walk, Barry actually took one of Ray's hands. There
was much less resistance from Barry when we left the Canteen
following our brief bit of shopping. I am a little puzzled by our
almost completely pleasant hour. I do not feel we have made this
much positive progress so I shall expect or at least not be sur-

prised to find the behavior of all not so agreeable tomorrow . . .
sure enough, it wasn't. Frank was much better, so rejoined us.
Barry was quite restless, eventually culminating in a tantrum.
Sociogram No. 3 indicates the degree of activity in the group.

As our group sessions continued the following progression
developed: A definite group structure was established. There is

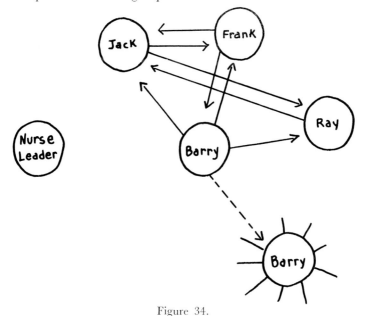

Figure 34.

togetherness, there is acceptance of one another and there is
definitely a feeling of responsibility for one another. The boys
are trying to place limitations on each other as though they were
doing some structuring of their group themselves. Although these
retarded children are dependent on leadership from the nursing
person in charge of them, they also tend to have a leader within
their group. Sociogram No. 4 indicates this activity.

I am becoming convinced that the retarded can definitely
profit from group therapy. Perhaps it will take much longer to
achieve maximum results as the retarded not only require a great
deal of conditioning in their learning but a lot of re-enforcement
in way of repetition before they feel secure in their situations. Any
age needs the understanding and reassurance of his peers which
can only be gained from small, comfortable and intimate group
situations.

We have been spending much time out-of-doors. I believe this is good since Nature is interesting with her wide variety of 'attention-getters.' Also, the boys are learning safe crossing of streets and the needs for limitations on their behavior if they

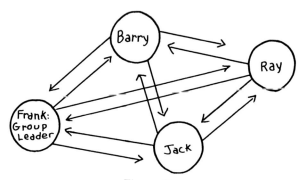

Figure 35.

are to venture into the community. By learning to set these limitations on themselves they are finding they are rewarded by new and more interesting experiences which they are learning to use as replacements for the old unacceptable behavior.

All our sessions are not successful; often I am forced to review the events of the day and must admit that though I tried very hard to hide my fatigue and shortness of patience, I remember the many methods of communication and without a doubt, I have communicated my 'problems of the day' in every gesture and tone of voice and have very likely left them feeling insecure and inattentive because of my attitude. It is well to always remember that the reactions of others are the product of our own action toward them.

Then, I am noticing that more and more we have very quiet but very pleasant sessions. Remember these four are a part of a very large group who for the most part are naturally very noisy; so at these times I make no effort to stimulate activity. . . . At times, when Ray screamed at me and hit me with his fist and the days when Barry would bite, strike at me, scream and throw his whole body around, I remember reading in Slav-son's works that a child therapist should be one whose adjust-ment to life was on the side of masochism . . .

All four members of the group are finally contributing to and receiving from the groups' efforts. The boys had learned to play together and disagree openly without inhibition or fear of rejection.

Then, a puzzling thing began to happen. Jack began to stray from the group. He didn't seem unhappy or angry, he would just wander away watching the others on the ground and it was clear his interests no longer were centered within the group. Not until I attended a ward team meeting and we were discussing group processes, and the social service member of the team ex-pressed a desire to take Jack for one-to-one therapy, did I sud-denly realize what was happening. I had become so group-cen-tered that I had forgotten that an individual only remains with a group as long as it fulfills his individual needs. Jack had out-grown his need of us! A startling fact. Our goal was being reached and I had not even realized it.

An evaluation of the progress of each other member of the group also showed progress.

Ray had developed an outlet for his inhibited feelings and was no longer withdrawn and passive.

Barry can run and play as free as the breeze without so much aggressiveness toward others. He has accepted personal contact in form of hand-holding and very noisy, tight 'bear-hugs.' During the 'bear-hugs' he lays his head against my chest and looks up without hesitancy or alarm reflected in his eyes; just content to have and accept human contact and no longer feel that it demands more of him than he can give.

Frank may seem pretty much the same on the surface; however, I remember that he has not rubbed his eye to gain attention nor felt the need to retreat to bed for almost two months. He also seems to have more respect for the wishes of the other patients on the ward and can understand their rights and limitations placed on his activities.

Our last session was of almost two hours duration, this in comparison to our beginning when it was hard to use a full hour in a constructive manner. I felt almost sorry that we were ter-minating our sessions and I don't think the boys have really be-lieved me when I keep telling them that we won't be going out as a group anymore. They are primarily interested with the present and what it has in store for them.

GROUP LEADERS OF PATIENT ACTIVITY PROGRAMS

Psychiatric treatment, to be effective, is a group process. It is a continuous process occurring on the wards, in industrial, recreational, occupational and many other activities and settings. It draws upon the skills of all of the members of the treatment team.

Psychiatric technician participation should not be limited only to ward activities. They can be assigned to supervise carefully se-

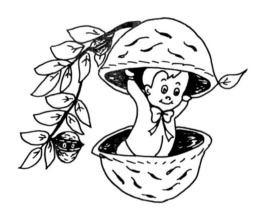

Figure 36. By permission of Marvel Baker, Psychiatric Technician, Sonoma State Hospital, Eldridge, California, and the Nursing Education Department of Sonoma State Hospital. Original poster created by Marvel Baker.

lected off-ward activities of a type not requiring the services of professionally trained specialists, craftsmen or industries personnel.

The activities may vary from diversional recreational activities, to the performance of useful tasks about the hospital which are beneficial to the hospital as a community, or a combination of both. In many cases the program could be of a pre-industrial nature. Tasks which provide training and motivation for the patients may be in farming, groundswork, maintenance, food service and other group activities. The effectiveness of the group should be measured in terms of patient improvement rather than in terms of economic gain to the hospital.

Objectives of such a developmental, or motivation, program include:

1. An outlet for physical aggression and development.
2. Provide opportunities for socialization through a variety of activities planned to meet the individual patient's needs.
3. Prevocational training.
4. Present opportunities for the development of accepted behavior patterns on a broader basis than is possible on the ward.
5. Provide a controlled situation in which the patient's ability to accept responsibility can be developed and evaluated.
6. To prevent regression and deterioration of the continued treatment (so-called chronic) patient.

Selection of patients for assignment to such a program would be made by the physician, if in his opinion the patient would improve through a highly motivated activities program. The range of selection can reach nearly all types of hospitalized individuals:

1. Both male and female.
2. Mentally retarded, moderate to mildly retarded range.
3. Mentally ill
   a. Closed ward patients needing close security provision.
   b. Emotionally disturbed or behavior problems.
   c. Acutely ill who have progressed to the point where they can be off the ward but still need close supervision.
   d. Regressed patient.
   e. Adolescent.
4. Both the skilled and the unskilled.

OBSERVATION AND RECORD KEEPING

Charting

Records must be maintained on patients for as long as they remain in a hospital. All forms used in the process of admitting a patient to a hospital, be it by voluntary admission or by court commitment, are kept in a master file. These in turn are usually maintained in a Medical Records room or storage space. Every patient is identified by name, case number, race, religion, sex and place of birth. This information accompanies him to any ward to which he may be transferred during his stay in the hospital.

The recording which the psychiatric technician must do is the charting at ward level. The purposes of keeping a chart are three fold:

1. To provide information about the patient for the doctor.
2. To provide a legal record of the patient's care and treatment.
3. To provide material which could supply useful information for future research studies.

The system of charting used will depend upon the hospital and the type of patients the hospital cares for. The small hospital or the hospital whose purpose is research oriented usually requires daily and detailed record keping. Large state hospitals which care for large numbers of patients who have been in residence for many years may require that only a monthly, or even only a quarterly, progress note be made on each patient. An exception may be made if a patient in such a hospital becomes acutely ill, which usually necessitates the transfer of the patient to the acute hospital or infirmary type ward within the hospital. Daily, more detailed charting is done during this period of acute illness.

PRINCIPLES FOR CHARTING

1. State what you have to say clearly, concisely and accurately. Do not use ten words to tell your story if five will say the same thing. Your charting of any specific activity of a patient should answer these six questions: Who? When? Where? What? How? Why?

2. Records must be legible and neat.
    a. Print or write clearly, using correct spelling and composition.
    b. Erasures are never permitted. The legality of a chart is destroyed if there is even a hint of an erasure on its pages. If an error *is* made on a record, the usual procedure followed is to draw a line through the error, print "error" and sign your full name. Example: error Mary Jones.
3. If abbreviations are called for, use only those which are standard.
4. All parts of the chart must be easily identified; i.e., the patient's name and case number must be entered in the appropriate space provided on each page.
5. The employee making an entry on a chart is usually required to sign his name, either in full or the first initial and last name.
6. The most important factors to observe and record pertaining to the patient are the behavior, appearance and activities in which he participates.

BEHAVIOR

This includes all types of actions: habits, dressing, eating, conversations, how he reacts to medications and treatments, how he relates with his fellow patients as well as to nursing personnel, any strange mannerisms and any seizures.

APPEARANCE

This includes what you see of the physical condition of the patient, a brief summary including:
1. Breath: pleasant or does he have halitosis?
2. Complexion: color, clearness, eruptions.
3. Eyes: clearness, expression, tearful.
4. Facial expressions: alert, bewildered, angry, happy, brooding, anxious, apprehensive.
5. Hair and condition of scalp: cleanliness, appearance, neat, tousled, sparse, dull, glossy.
6. Locomotion: walking, wheelchair, crawling, bedfast.
7. Nutrition of body: emaciated, well-nourished, obese.
8. Perspiration: entire body, or portions, day or night.

9. Pulse: rate, rhythm, quality.
10. Respiration: rate, rhythm, quality, coughing, hiccoughing.
11. Skin: cleanliness, general condition, warm, cold, color, tone.
12. Stools and urine: frequency, color, discomfort, anything abnormal.
13. Vomiting: if present, amount, color, consistency, material.

ACTIVITIES

This includes all hospital activities in which the patient is included. The activity may be medical, such as a visit to a dental clinic or a laboratory test; it may be social, such as a dance or it may be an industrial therapy assignment, to list just a few.

CHARTING AIDS

A few abbreviations which are helpful in accurate charting are:

Times

q.d.	—every day	p.c.	—after meals
b.i.d.	—2 times a day	h.s.	—bedtime
t.i.d.	—3 times a day	stat	—at once
q.i.d.	—4 times a day	p.r.n.	—when required
q.h.	—every hour	ad. lib.	—at pleasure
a.c.	—before meals		

Measurements

Gm.	—gram	z	—dram
mg.	—milligram	oz. or ʒ	—ounce
gr.	—grain	gtt	—drop
min.	—minim	tsp.	—teaspoon
c.c.	—cubic centimeter	ss	—one-half

Other Symbols You Should Recognize

A.M.	—morning	q s.	—quantity sufficient
B.M.	—bowel movement	tbc. or	—tuberculosis;
B.P.	—blood pressure	t.b.	tubercle bacillus
c	—with	EEG	—electroencephalogram
C	—centigrade	T.P.R.	—temperature, pulse, respiration
EKG	—electrocardiogram	Wt.	—weight
H$_2$O	—water	WBC or	—white blood count or
I.M.	—intramuscular	wbc	cells
IV.	—intravenous	RBC or	—red blood count or
O$_2$	—oxygen	rbc	cells
s	—without		

Vocabulary

Semantics, or the study of the meaning of words, especially those used in psychiatry, can easily become extremely time consuming. It is advisable for a psychiatric technician to become well acquainted with the use of a medical dictionary, Webster's dictionary and a student's dictionary of psychological terms, in the course of his studies and work in psychiatric nursing.

However, you should become familiar with some of the more commonly used terms so that you will know what the psychiatrist, and other treatment personnel, are talking about when they discuss a patient's behavior.

First of all, who's doing the talking about what:

Psychiatrist: A medical doctor who specializes in psychiatry. He has an M.D. degree.

Psychiatry: A basic medical science which deals with the beginnings, diagnosis, prevention and treatment of emotional illness and unsatisfactory behavior. It is particularly concerned with what causes abnormal thought, behavior and symptoms.

Psychology: A nonmedical branch of science which deals with the study of mental processes and behavior.

Psychologist: Is not a physician or M.D. The psychologist may hold a Master's degree or a Ph.D. (Doctor of Philosophy) in psychology.

Now for some of the words:

Affect: Any specific kind of feeling or emotion especially when it is attached to a particular person or object.

Ambivalence: The presence of two opposing desires or emotions, at the same time, toward the same person, object or goal. Example: Wanting to do two different things at the same time.

Compulsions: These are actions which often result in a ritual or which occur in an automatic fashion without the subject being able to control them.

Delusions: False beliefs which cannot be changed by logical argument and reasoning and which often bear no relation to the individual's educational and cultural background. The most common types are:

    1. Hypochondriacal delusions: The patient has distorted ideas of disordered bodily functions, such as the body rotting away or obstruction of the bowels. (A patient once told me in all seriousness that he had "triple bowel obstruction," yet all the while he was busily working on the ward.)

2. Feelings of passivity: The patient expresses feelings of being under control of some external force, such as xray or the radio.
3. Ideas of reference: The patient thinks he is being watched and spied upon, or that he is being talked about.
4. Paranoid ideas: Ideas that people and things are working against the patient.
5. Grandiose delusions: Vary from an increased self confidence in a patient to frank, expansive delusions (such as the patient who was going to fire all the employees at a hospital and hire an entire new "crew.")

Dynamics: How a behavior pattern develops.

Empathy: A feeling or sharing of felings with another person, this being a deeper and closer feeling than that of sympathy.

Hallucinations: This is an imaginary sensory perception which is unrelated to any external stimulation. They occur as:
1. Visual (sight)—may see a vision or some unusual picture in front of the eyes.
2. Auditory (hearing)—may be called by name (when alone) or may hear strange noises.
3. Olfactory (smell)—patient may think he smells strange odors or smells.
4. Gustatory (taste)—patient may complain of a peculiar taste in the mouth.
5. Tactile—patient may complain of strange and peculiar skin sensations.

Illusions: Misinterpretations of sensory impressions. An example: A shadow is considered a real man.

Insight: The degree of understanding which the individual may or may not have in regards to his illness and how it affects his behavior and thinking.

Mood: State of mind of the individual especially as it is affected by emotion. It is closely related to "affect," just lasting longer.

Obsessions: Recurring thoughts in the mind of the patient. The thoughts are of an unpleasant intruding nature and the patient is not free to think of anything else.

Phobias: Feelings of fear which alter the outward behavior of the individual. Phobias may so influence the person's life that he will look for procedures which will avoid the fear-producting situation, such as crowds, or food, or darkness, and may deeply affect the person's life.

Psychosomatic: A term which indicates the importance of the interaction of the mind (psyche) and the body (soma) and how one is dependent upon the other in regards to the physical and emotional aspects of a person.

Rapport: The establishment of a harmonious relationship between two or more people.

Remission: A period of lessening of the symptoms of the disease. Differs from "cure" in that recurrence is to be expected.

A CASE STUDY

One method of becoming better acquainted with the techniques used in caring for patients is through a plan of individualized patient observation and care. The aims of such a study could be all, or any part, of the following:

1. To realize the need for understanding each patient as an individual in order to appreciate his problems and outlook.
2. To be aware of the significance of the preventive aspects of nursing.
3. To learn to collect information about the patient with tact and skill.
4. To be able to work out a nursing plan to fit the needs of the individual patient on the basis of his special problems.
5. To record nursing observations in an organized, systematic way.

That such a plan can be effective is best demonstrated by the story of a real little girl as observed, cared for and recorded by a real psychiatric technician.

From the record of the preadmission (to the hospital) interview which was done by a social service worker, I learned that the situation in Mary Doe's home was almost impossible. The father had recently had a heart attack and could work only part time. There were three other children besides Mary, she being the youngest. Her mother had stated: 'Mary was destructive, aggressive, extremely hyperactive and was not toilet trained, but would have her bowel movement in the corner of the room. She would not wear clothing. Sometimes Mary would have forty to fifty seizures a week some lasting as long as 4 hours at a time. I kept Mary locked in a room because she would run away if given the chance.'

So, at the age of five and a half Mary Doe was admitted to the state hospital. The first two years of her stay at the hospital was not on my ward, but her chart showed that she had many problems of adjustment, such as her diet, to many new and strange people and to medicines used to control her seizures. She was also started on a toilet training routine. During the third year of her stay at the hospital Mary was transferred to my ward and during the remainder of that year and the next, because she had so many continuous seizures, it was necessary for her to be transferred into the Acute Medical ward a total of seventy times. Then a new routine was established by the doctor for Mary's medicines. And for two years several of the technicians remained constant on my ward, including myself.

We had observed that Mary apparently enjoyed the excitement and attention which she received when having seizures. After discussing this with the doctor, the policy of the nursing personnel was to take it all in a calm, seemingly off-hand manner, but even though Mary is not aware of it, she *was* being observed. She is urged to sit down and be quiet and often that is all that is needed. If she continues to show symptoms of an impending seizure she is given her medicine in her food at meal time. Sometimes she has one seizure during the day and occasionally two, but has not gone into continuous seizures for two years.

Mary likes to help the technicians around the ward. She especially likes to help the night shift people. She likes to drag bundles of sheets to the laundry room door. There is never any heavily soiled sheets in the bundle and she just catches hold of the corners of the bundle to drag it to the laundry room door. If allowed to do this she is happy. She likes to be told 'That's a good girl, Mary.' Whenever she is denied the chance to do this task, she becomes angry and frustrated, and despite any efforts of the nursing personnel, has a seizure. It is hoped that in the near future Mary can help with dressing other patients or in some way substitute for this activity and still feel wanted and needed.

Mary is healthy and happy on my ward but she cannot adjust to changes very well. After she passed her tenth birthday she was transferred to another ward to see if she could take part in a more advanced training program. But she developed such upset behavior, as tearing up her clothing, running away from the ward and having more frequent seizures, that in less than two months she was transferred back to my ward.

She has improved so much over her former behavior that she now goes to church services, to the movies and on bus rides. She goes out walking and plays outside on the grass with other patients when the weather is nice. She has a favorite playmate, Susie, and they play together for long periods at a time.

Mary understands but cannot carry on a conversation. She can make a four or five word sentence. She points out objects and names them. Once, when on a bus ride, she pointed to a windmill and said 'Windmill?' another time she noticed the ward's sewing machine and said 'sewing machine?' She makes a statement out of a question.

Mary is given medicines on a regular three times a day schedule for control of her seizures and there is also an order medicine to be given if definite symptoms of seizure appear.

Mary's family never visit but since she does not expect it she does not seem to let it matter too much. I guess we are her family.

Patient Observation by a Psychiatric Technician

B. L. was born on September 13, 1949, and the pregnancy of the mother was presumably normal as was the delivery, but B. L. did weigh a large amount at birth (ten pounds and three ounces).

At the age of two years, B. L. was thrown from a moving car and was knocked unconscious. This left a bruise on the right frontal area of her head which has now turned into a small lump. Bedrest for a few days was the recommendation of their family doctor. I find nothing stating that this accident had anything to do with her retardation.

At four years of age, B. L.'s parents tried to get her into

school but she was rejected. Later in the special class in the first grade she caused quite a disturbance in doing such things as tearing displays from the blackboard. She was very possessive of her teacher and got jealous when the teacher showed special attention to other students.

At four years of age, B. L.'s mother and father were divorced. Her father remarried.

B. L. stayed with her mother and two other siblings, but B. L. became mean to the other two children. Her mother decided B. L. needed more help than she could give, and so requested admission to the State Hospital in December of 1957. When this happened the father and step-mother intervened, stating the child was not retarded, that all she needed was a little love and affection.

The father and step-mother then took B. L. to live with them. They redecorated her room and bought her a complete new wardrobe. They seemed to be very happy to have B. L. living with them for they had no children of their own and were thinking seriously about adopting a child. B. L. was just what they were looking for, but as time went by, B. L. presented quite a problem in their home. It seems the more attention she received, the more she demanded. She was quite possessive of her step-mother, even requesting that she not speak to other people.

Believing that B. L. needed more special care than they could give her, they interviewed the foster home. Since the home had five other children they felt it would not be of any gain for B. L. so they contacted the State Hospital. They felt she needed the psychiatric help that the hospital could give.

The step-mother once said "I want to run when I see her face coming out of the bedroom in the morning." She also stated that the child had an abnormal interest in sex, which she expressed in speech only.

The father stated that both the mother and the step-mother had threatened to commit suicide because of the extreme problems B. L. presented but later apologized for saying this.

One doctor stated that most of B. L.'s problem was because of the emotional conflict in her family.

Then B. L. was put up for admission and admission was granted immediately because the father had threatened to kill the mother.

So, at the age of eight and one-half years, B. L. was admitted to the State Hospital as moderately retarded with an I.Q. of 54 due to defective fetal development.

This child was first recommended to ward A where at first she was very shy and retiring. Later, as she became adjusted to her strange surroundings, she became more out-going, although she did seem to be inclined to have one "best friend" at a time.

Two years later B. L. was transferred to ward B. She acted somewhat the same as she did on ward A. She was shy at first and later became more forward as she became adjusted to the ward.

B. L. participates in all off-ward activities such as: dances, shows, church, special programs, parties, and many other activities. She is under the Industrial Therapy program and is also active in the Friendship Service. She is found to be very cooperative and sweet in the activities held by the Rehabilitation Services. She obviously enjoys and does very well in all activities.

While on ward A, B. L. attended the summer camp in the mountains. The child was very thrilled at this, as were her parents. At summer camp she was found very cooperative and took care of all her personal needs.

Now she is enrolled in school at the hospital where she does quite well. Of course, considering the change into the school program, she exhibited her usual shyness but later adjusted very well. In school, she is quite capable of solving her own problems and tries to do what is asked of her.

B. L. has a speech defect of infantile sounds such as "dis" for "this" but it is believed that with age she will out-grow this defect.

An outstanding interest of B. L.'s, in which she participates, is chorus. She was very regular in attendance and learns lyrics very fast.

While on A, she was recommended for a special academic class in which she now participates.

In her appearance, B. L. is a normal appearing, pretty blonde, with blue eyes and a very winning smile. She is quite neat for a twelve-year-old girl. She still has this lisp, but as stated before, she seems to be out-growing it. She was quite obese when first admitted to the hospital but is now growing into a quite tall and rather slender girl.

I have noticed that she speaks of having a "boy friend," she does not discuss him freely with me. She still is inclined to have one "best-friend."

Her parents come to see her very often. She seems to enjoy their visits and appears to be quite fond of her family, especially her father.

B. L. has not had any outstanding illnesses since her admittance to the hospital. This child has no need for any kind of medication.

B. L. seems to be progressing nicely in every respect. She is quite pleasant and a joy to have around. She can be trusted, is able to hold an interesting conversation and is well liked by everyone on the ward.

Post-script: After two and a half years B. L. left the State Hospital, not to her parents, but to a foster mother and foster home care, where she is reported to be doing very well.

Chapter V

MENTAL ILLNESS

HISTORICAL BACKGROUND

The humane care of the mentally ill has taken many centuries to reach its present day level of understanding of the sick mind.

In the middle ages the mentally sick person was thought to be possessed by demons or evil spirits and were treated accordingly. The procedures usually involved some type of religious ceremony in which the evil spirits were driven from the sick person's body. Physical punishment and torture of the patient played an important part in the "treatment."

During the seventeenth and eighteenth centuries the insane were chained in dungeons and forgotten by all except the dungeon keeper. Very few of these inmates ever lived to return to society. It was during the last decade of the eighteenth century that Philippe Pinel, in France, removed the chains from a patient who had been so restrained for forty years in the Bicetre, a Paris institution. Pinel was the first of many who have campaigned to eliminate the use of mechanical restraint in the treatment of the mentally ill. In England more humane treatment of mentally ill patients was made possible through the work of William Tuke and his brother. They were responsible for the founding of the York Retreat. The Pennsylvania Hospital was finished in 1756 in America and it was here that Dr. Benjamin Rush initiated many concepts of humane treatment of the mentally ill, including the use of occupational therapy. Dr. Rush was the first American doctor to write a book on mental disorders. He is known as the "Father of American Psychiatry."

Prior to the middle of the nineteenth century there were no special institutions for the care of the mentally ill or mentally deficient. They were "put away" in either the poorhouse or in the jails. No consideration was given to the respect and dignity of the individual. No attempt was made at segregation or classification. If the individuals were only mildly demented or deficient but had strong backs, they were in many instances sold to the highest bidder, for servants and cheap labor.

But in 1841, in a day when it was unheard of for a woman to do anything outside of her home except perhaps to teach school, Dorothy Lynde Dix dared to be different. Never physically very strong, at the age of forty years she started a reform movement which she continued for the remainder of her life, for the better treatment of the insane. She was instrumental in so arousing the public's interest that many states built hospitals and provided treatment and care for the mentally ill. She played an important part in the founding of the St. Elizabeth's Hospital in Washington, D.C., as well as initiating reforms in other countries. Some writers describe her as the "Apostle of the Insane."

As the years went by more and more state hospitals were built for the care of the mentally ill. The majority of these institutions were built in a location away from the town or city, which in turn encouraged the image, in the mind of the average person, of the mentally sick person as being one who was dangerous and not safe to be outside of barred walls.

It was not until after the beginning of the twentieth century that thought was given to what might be done to recognize the early stages of the various mental conditions and what could be done to prevent them from developing. In 1907 Clifford Beers, who had been mentally ill and a patient in various institutions himself, wrote the book *The Mind That Found Itself*. As a result of his own experiences he was aroused to the need for educating and training the public in the field of mental hygiene. In 1908 he organized the first State Society for Mental Hygiene, in Connecticut, and one year later the first National Committee was organized under his direction. The Mental Hygiene movement has become well known not only in the United States but in other countries as well, its activities pertaining to normal human beings as much as to the abnormal.

At about the same time that the Mental Hygiene movement was getting under way, Sigmund Freud in Europe was developing new theories as to the dynamics, or the driving forces, of the unconscious mind of an individual. The methods of treatment grouped under the term "psychotherapy" resulted from his work.

Many physical and medical agents were also introduced for treating mental illnesses. One of the first was the use of malaria fever therapy in 1917, for the treatment of the mental condition which results from the infection of the central nervous system by syphilis. In the 1930's many discoveries were made pertaining to the miracles which could be worked by the use of vitamins. It was proven that many of the delirious and confused mental conditions which occur in such diseases as pellegra and alcoholism could be cured by the administration of vitamins.

The use of various types of shock therapies came upon the scene of battle against mental illness in 1933, the use of insulin first being introduced by Manfred Sakel in Vienna, Austria. Two years later Von Meduna, in Budapest, Hungary, first used metrazol to produce convulsive shock therapy; this in turn to be followed by the use of electric shock therapy, or E.S.T. as it was commonly called.

The next attack made against mental illness was in the form of psychosurgery, or surgical procedures performed on the brain. Prefrontal lobotomy was the operation most commonly used, the technic first used in the United States in 1936 by Drs. Freeman and Watts.

The most recent weapon used in the struggle for mental health is the tranquilizer drugs. It is early yet to say that these drugs produce lasting effects; suffice it to say that during the past five years the rate of release of patients from state hospitals has continued to increase throughout the nation.

As our scientists go ever forward in the exploration of outer space, so too will scientists continue to explore the mysteries of the mind and to seek the reasons for its going "out of orbit."

Chapter VI

PRESENT DAY FACTS ABOUT
MENTAL ILLNESS

THERE is a real bell behind the bell symbol of the National Association for Mental Health. (The sign of the ringing bell has become the symbol of the fight against mental illness.) It weighs 300 pounds and was cast from chains and shackles once used to restrain mental patients. The metal was melted down on April 13, 1953, in Baltimore. On the bell is inscribed these words:

Cast from shackles which bound them,
this bell shall ring out hope for the
mentally ill and victory over mental
illness.

THE EXTENT OF MENTAL ILLNESS

At least one person in every ten—19,000,000 people in all—has some form of mental or emotional illness (from mild to severe) that needs psychiatric treatment.

Mental illness is known to be an important factor in many physical illnesses, even heart disease and tuberculosis.

At least 50 per cent of all the millions of medical and surgical cases treated by private doctors and hospitals have a mental illness complication.

HOW MANY ENTER AND LEAVE MENTAL HOSPITALS?

There are more people in hospitals with mental illness, at any one time, than with all other diseases combined, including cancer, heart disease, tuberculosis and every other killing and crippling disease.

Last year about 1,100,000 persons received treatment in our public, federal and private mental hospitals and in the psychiatric wards of general hospitals. (This included the patients who were in the hospitals at the beginning of the year, plus those who were admitted during the year.)

On any one day of the year about 760,000 persons are under the psychiatric care of these hospitals, including about 149,000 who are not actually in the hospital but are on "trial visit" or a similar form of supervision.

Each year about 600,000 persons are admitted for psychiatric treatment in mental hospitals and in the psychiatric sections of general hospitals. Of these, over 100,000 are admitted for the second or third time.

In spite of the increase in the number of patients treated during the year in state and county mental hospitals, fewer patients were in the hospital at the end of the year than at the beginning. In 1963 the resident hospital population declined again, slightly, for an eighth successive year.

WHAT ARE CHANCES OF LEAVING A MENTAL HOSPITAL?

With good care and treatment, at least seven of ten patients can leave mental hospitals partially or totally recovered.

Data from a number of states show that about 75 per cent of those admitted for the first time leave the hospital within the first year.

In the case of the most prevalent mental crippler, schizophrenia, the chances of recovery or improvement have jumped from about 20 per cent to about 80 per cent in the last forty years. The higher rate occurs, however, only when proper treatment is administered.

In the case of two other serious mental illnesses, involutional psychosis and maniac depressive psychosis, the chances of recovery or improvement are about 65 per cent and 75 per cent respectively.

In the past, readmission rates have been as high as 35 per cent of the patients discharged within a year. Recent research has shown that this figure can be reduced to about 10 per cent with continuing and thorough rehabilitation service, including medical, social and vocational after-care.

ILLNESSES AND AGES OF MENTAL HOSPITAL PATIENTS

New patients admitted to public (state and county) hospitals fall principally into the following diagnoses and approximate age groups:

Schizophrenia: About 23 per cent of new patients are schizophrenics: most of these fall between fifteen and thirty-four years of age. They make up about 50 per cent of the resident population of mental hospitals, because of their youth on admission and long-term hospitalization.

Senile brain disease and cerebral arteriosclerosis: These psychoses account for about 21 per cent of new admissions, usually over the age of sixty-five. Because of high death rates among these patients, they represent only about 13 per cent of the hospital population.

Involutional psychosis: About 3.5 per cent of new patients admitted to mental hospitals; usually between the ages of forty-five and sixty-five.

Manic-depressive and psychotic depressive reactions: About 3.5 per cent of new admissions, usually between thirty-five and fifty-five.

Alcohol intoxication and alcohol addiction: About 14.7 per cent of new admissions; usually between twenty-five and fifty-five.

Personality disorders other than alcoholism: About 8.5 per cent of new admissions; between fifteen and thirty-five.

Other disorders, each of low incidence, make up 26 per cent of new admissions.

MENTAL ILLNESS AMONG CHILDRED AND YOUNG ADULTS

Mental illness occurs at all ages, including childhood.

It is estimated that there are more than half a million mentally ill children in the United States classified as psychotic or borderline cases. Most of these children are suffering from the psychiatric disorder known as childhood schizophrenia.

Only a very small percentage of the total are receiving any kind of psychiatric treatment.

About 23,000 children and young adults, with serious mental disorders, are admitted as patients to public mental hospitals each year. Four thousand are under fifteen, and 19,000 between fifteen and twenty-four.

On any one day in the year, there are 26,500 children and young adults with serious mental disorders, in our mental hospitals. Four thousand, five hundred are under fifteen, and 22,000 are between fifteen and twenty-four.

Conservatively estimated, an additional 271,000 children under eighteen are served in psychiatric clinics each year, for less severe mental disorders.

MENTAL HOSPITAL FACILITIES

Number of Hospitals

There are 600 mental hospitals in the United States. They include 288 state and county hospitals, forty neuropsychiatric hospitals of the Veterans Administration, three other federal hospitals and 259 private hospitals.

In addition, there are 128 public and 209 private institutions for the mentally defective.

Approximately 600 general hospitals, or about 11 per cent of the total number, have separate units for treating psychiatric patients. An additional number, estimated at about 200, treat psychiatric patients in their regular medical facilities.

MAINTENANCE COSTS

The average cost of caring for each patient in public mental hospitals is $5.11 per day or $2,120.00 per year. One state spends as little as $2.84 per patient per day. The top figure is $10.80.

By comparison, general hospitals spend more than $35 per day per patient. Veterans Administration psychiatric hospitals spend a little more than $14 per day.

COST OF MENTAL ILLNESS

About $1,788,000,000 is spent annually on the care and treatment of patients in state, county and federal mental hospitals.

Expenditures for community mental health services during 1962 totaled $93,800,000 (compared to $25,800,000 in 1956.)*

---

*From: 1964 Fact Sheet, issued by the National Association for Mental Health, 10 Columbus Circle, New York 19, N. Y. by permission of: George Argys, Executive Director, California Association for Mental Health, Sacramento 14, California.

Chapter VII

MENTAL HEALTH

Mental health is something all of us want for ourselves whether we know it by name or not. When we speak of happiness, or peace of mind, or satisfaction, we are usually talking about mental health. But mental health is far more than merely the absence of mental illness. The state of one's mental health is one of the most important factors which influences the events of everyone's daily living. It means the over-all way that people get along everywhere: in their family, at school, on the job, at play, with their fellowman and with the community in which they live. A person is said to be mentally healthy if he can adjust to new situations, meet all emotional and physical needs without undue stress and still have some energy left, as well as the desire, to contribute constructively to his society.

However, no one can escape stress. There are varying degrees and forms of stress all of which have some impact upon the individual's health. Stress has been defined by one authority as the "rate of all wear and tear" caused by life. All emotions such as love or hate involve stress. The emotional stress that most affects one is the kind that makes it difficult or nearly impossible to relax; feelings of frustration, fear, anger or worry which one may bottle up inside one's self can be injurious to both the physical and mental health. It is the unduly intense and persistent emotions which lead to most of the trouble. On the other hand no one would want to exist as an automaton without feeling; it is important to know that emotions themselves are good for us. Knowing and accepting one's physical and emotional limitations is an individual's first step to understanding of self and those around them. Relationships with others is more satisfying as a result of acquiring such understanding.

There are many ways by which people have learned to handle tensions successfully and to weather the rough spots of life more smoothly. Some of the following suggestions may help you or someone close to you.

WAYS TO HANDLE TENSIONS

"Balance work with play: That old saying about all work and no play making Jack a dull boy still makes sense. Besides, all work may also give Jack an ulcer or harm his health in other ways! If Jack— or Jill—has trouble taking it easy long enough to get some fun out of life, he probably ought to schedule time for recreation. For many people, an interesting hobby can be relaxing as well as constructive. On the other hand, work can occasionally be a kind of "cure" for emotional situations that are hard to bear—like the death of a loved one, a divorce, or the breaking of an engagement. Getting busy helps some people to stop stewing about their troubles.

"Loaf a little: Very active people who feel guilty about occasionally just sitting and doing plain nothing ought to give themselves a chance to learn the art of loafing. While too much inactivity breeds boredom and may even cause stress, a few minutes a day of doing nothing may help us to tackle our work with renewed enthusiasm.

"Put off until tomorrow: Some people need to learn to let some things go. When a work load seems overwhelming, remember you can do only one task at a time. Concentrate on the particular job at hand and then go on to the next one without worrying about everything that has to be done. Some things can almost always be set aside until later, or until tomorrow. And work usually goes faster and smoother when you have this attitude of doing one thing at a time.

"Work off tensions: When we're upset or angry, we can try to blow off steam or work off our feelings with physical exercise. Pitching into some activity, like working in the garden, taking a long walk, playing a game of tennis or going in for some other sport, not only helps to relieve anger but makes it easier to face and handle irritating problems more calmly.

"Talk out troubles: It helps to "get it off your chest" sometimes by

confiding worries to a sympathetic friend. When what appears to be a serious problem starts to get you down, it's wise to discuss it with your clergyman or family doctor, or with an understanding member of your own family. Often another person can help you to get your feelings into focus and to see your problems in a new light. If your problems seem to be getting out of hand, your own doctor may want to recommend a specialist, or refer you to a guidance clinic or a family service agency.

"Learn to accept: What you cannot change. Many of us get upset about circumstances which are beyond our control. Sometimes we even try to make people over to suit our own ideals and then feel frustrated or let down when we find that this cannot be done. We can look for the best in others while realizing that nobody is faultless.

"Get away from it all: When you feel that you are going around in circles with a problem or worry, try to divert yourself. As simple a thing as going to the movies, reading a story, or visiting a friend can help to get you out of a rut. And there's no harm in running away from a painful situation long enough to catch your breath and regain the composure you need to come back and face the problem. When possible and practical, a brief trip, a change of scene, can give you new perspective. There are times when we all need to "escape"—even if it's just a respite from routine.

"Have regular checkups: It's important to go to your doctor or clinic for periodic checkups. Just as the mind affects the body's working order, physical condition affects a person's outlook on life. If you keep yourself physically fit you'll have more zest for living and be able to take stress and handle tensions more easily.

"But there are no easy ways nor simple solutions to the problem of life which cause undue stress and tension. Some of the ideas you read can be useful. Experience, too, is a teacher. And other people can be helpful. By making the effort, we often find new and better ways to deal with the tensions of our lives."*

There is no clean-cut line that neatly divides the mentally healthy from the unhealthy. There are many different degrees of mental health but these degrees cannot be measured on a thermometer, as

---

*Metropolitan Life Insurance Company: *Stress and What It Means to You.* New York, 1964.

degrees of heat are measured, but rather as shades of grey, none being all white or all black. As Dr. Will Menninger stated on a nationally televised discussion on February 25, 1962, the state of person's mental health "may fluctuate from a deep grey to a bright white." No one characteristic by itself can be taken as evidence of good mental health, nor the lack of anyone as evidence of mental illness. Nobody has all the traits of good mental health all the time. The measure of a person's emotional stability is the degree to which he can adapt to life situations. Most of us have had the experience of "being in the dumps" or having said "I've sure got the blues today," as well as having had the experience of tackling the problems of the day with a feeling of elation. A prolonged period of feeling "blue" or of feeling "elated" would be abnormal behavior as is evidenced in some mental illnesses.

The type of acceptance or rejection of an individual's behavior, especially if the behavior strays from what is considered normal, is determined by the community and society in which the individual lives. It is unfortunate that in this enlightened age there are many members of our society who look upon an individual who is mentally ill as one who is "insane" and who should "be locked up where he can't hurt anyone." However, great progress has been made in a relatively few years in the education of the general public to an awareness of and an understanding and acceptance of mental illnesses. The maiden lady living alone in the country who is heard talking loudly, with no one else in sight, and is seen throwing the kitchen pots and pans against the walls, is spoken of in an understanding tone as "anyone who lives alone has the right to talk to themselves." If the same lady lived in a crowded city apartment building, such behavior would no doubt be reported to the police, if for no other reason than that of disturbing the peace.

The process of learning how to understand, observe and interpret the behavior of human beings is complicated not only by the fact that they are not like peas in a pod, but the individual's own personal life experiences.

Chapter VIII

WHAT CAUSES MENTAL ILLNESS?

THERE is no one specific cause for a person to become mentally ill. Gone forever is the notion that the mentally ill person is an exception. The behavior and/or the feelings of a person which leads him to either seek help voluntarily or causes his family to seek help for him is but a symptom of some underlying causative agent, be it physical or mental. The body and mind cannot be separated and put into neat little compartments when searching for the cause of mental illness. Old labels no longer fit. The *whole* person: not only his personality, but his heredity, his physical structure, his health both mental and physical, his emotional attitude toward life, all must be taken into consideration before a diagnosis can be made. The process of arriving at a diagnosis has gradually become a matter of understanding the way in which an individual has been taken with a disability, partly self-imposed and partly externally brought about. However, the fundamental determining factors of mental health and illness are the same in every walk of life. The culture and income and education account for whether the individual will handle his problem, whether he understands himself as sick, whether he seeks help and so on.

Changes in the brain due to the processes of aging, or to injury to the head, or to tumors, or to diseases which damage the brain tissue, or excessive use of alcohol or drugs of certain kinds are some of the organic, or physical, causes of mental illnesses. Even when there is some such obvious reason for a mental illness, the behavior shown by the individual may be but an exaggeration of the way he has always behaved; that is, if he has always been a 'lone wolf' type he may become very withdrawn and depressed. The behavior of a woman who has a 'mental breakdown' when going through the 'change of life' or menopause is not due merely to the fact that her reproductive glands will no longer be functioning. Deeper emotional problems are involved. If she is a spinster it may mean to her an end of any hope for love and romance. If she has always been a 'worrier' and has always been overly fussy about everything she does, she may become extremely agitated as well as depressed.

However, the majority of mental illnesses have no physical reason for their occurrence. The illness may be considerd as the response of an individual to a situation of overwhelming stress with which he cannot cope. No two authorities will give exactly the same causes for any one mental illness but in general it will be pinpointed to a situation which has created a conflict with resulting anxiety within the individual. The immediate reason which may be given as causing the mental break may be the death of a loved one or a failure in business. Many times the illness may occur suddenly with no apparent warning signs, when in reality the individual for years has been like a volcano inside, literally boiling with hidden fears, hatreds or anxieties. The entire life of the person must be thoroughly explored before he can be helped because the seeds of his anxieties may have been sown before he ever learned to walk.

Mental illness should be looked upon as a way of behaving and not as a "thing." It should not be over-simplified but neither is it a secretive, weird or unhuman condition. We all know what it is from our own experiences. Actually, the expressions coming from everyday life such as "I feel as if I were going to pieces" or "I'm so nervous and upset" are often more accurate than the technical words and do not have the same dreadful implications. We may become a bit demoralized, or even make some serious mistakes, but we fight against it and do the best we can. Whenever a person reaches such a mental state he needs help, not a "label."

As was stated in an earlier chapter, the pattern of development of an individual's personality is set in earliest childhood. The child who is wanted from the day he is conceived, whose parents are genuinely fond of him without being over-protective; who, when needing discipline can depend upon its being fair and consistent, and whose quest for growth and independence is not unduly restricted by his parents, is well on the way to developing into a mentally healthy adult. On the other hand, the child whose mother is over-anxious, is aggressive, is over-protective, and who on one day would smother the youngster with love and next day would not want him near her, may become so emotionally upset that psychiatric aid will be needed before he reaches his teens.

The recent advances in our knowledge suggests quite strongly that the mental health of an individual is linked in many ways with the social interaction which takes place in the family group. The relationships between the father and mother are reflected in the child. The manner in which a child will learn to respond to the authority figure in his family will set the pattern for his behavior toward society. In the 'good' home environment a boy will identify with the father and the father will think of the boy proudly as "just like his old man." For the mother the boy is not a rival for her husband's love but is regarded as a recreation of the man she loves and admires. In a similar manner, a girl will pattern herself after her mother. If there is emotional conflict between the parents the child will become confused and be harmed psychologically because regardless of the parent chosen as a model, the affection and approval of the other parent will be lacking.

A child should be permitted to be dependent and demanding in early life, becoming independent as they grow older and gain confidence. Even with this "permission" the successful parent gives the youngster a feeling of security by establishing controls for standards of behavior. Even a very young child needs a "pillar of strength" to turn to for guidance. How he learns the "do's" and "don'ts" of social living will relate directly to the type of adult which he becomes. Any of the training processes, such as toilet training, will create rewards and punishments (the good and the bad). This will usually cause the child to have feelings of uncertainty in regards to his relationships with his parents. He doesn't know whether to hate them or to love them. It is best if the training processes are performed in such a way that love, not hate, will develop.

If a child has to "grow up" and assume responsibilities which are too great for him too soon in life, he develops feelings of resentment which result in poor adjustments to life, in some instances progressing to anti-social behavior. Non-organization in social relationships usually results from poor discipline in childhood. Hostility and aggressiveness are traits of non-organization for which society pays a high penalty. There is a difference between hostility and aggression, hostility being passive while aggression is active. Hostility is a pattern of emotion and may be born of resentment. Aggression is a pattern of behavior and may follow feelings of hostility.

On the other hand, the child who clings to dependency and is not encouraged to give up his childish ways, is on the way to becoming a neurotic, poorly adjusted adult. A balance between the two patterns will usually result in a reasonably well-adjusted adult.

Chapter IX

PATTERNS OF ADJUSTMENT

Everything that you see in life, you see in
The mirror of your mind.
And if your mind be warped or cloudy,
So shall the image of what you see be
Warped or cloudy.*

THE process of living is one of constant struggle between the needs and desires of the individual and other forces which hamper and frustrate him. This produces anxiety, which the average normal person attempts to relieve in one of three ways:

1. He can refuse to face them.
2. He can fight back.
3. He can compromise.

In the process of compromising, the individual will use various patterns of adjustment, or mental mechanisms. The person's mind erects these "defenses" to assist him in arriving at some sort of a solution which will relieve the pain and tension caused by a particular conflict. The mentally healthy, as well as the mentally ill person, uses these mental mechanisms but the mentally well-adjusted individual just doesn't find it necessary to use them as often.

Definitions and interpretations of the adjustive techniques vary with an author's opinion. However, the following figures† present a visual image which will aid the student to more easily understand the meaning of each term.

All of these patterns of behavior may be used by any of us throughout our life time. Perhaps you can recognize yourself and thereby be better able to understand and help others. These compromises when used to any great degree may be considerd a warning of serious maladjustment to life. After all, it is not always the

---

*Townshend, Frank: *Earth*. New York, Alfred A. Knopf, Inc., 1929.

†Created by E. J. Rice, Sr. Psychiatric Technician II, Porterville State Hospital, Porterville, California.

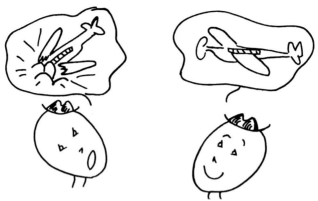

REPRESSION: He saw an airplane crash which so shocked him that he has unconsciously forgotten that he ever saw it happen and sees the plane as it was before the accident occurred.

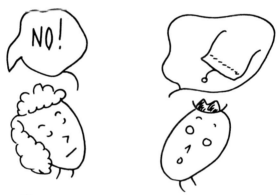

SUPPRESSION: Her refusal to go out with him is painful so he unconsciously 'pulls the shade' and refuses to think about it.

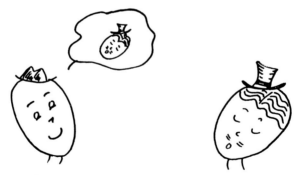

IDENTIFICATION: He has identified so closely with his favorite handsome movie actor that this is the way he sees himself.

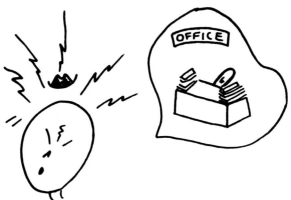

CONVERSION: He cannot face all the overdue work waiting for him at the office so he develops a headache so intense that he is unable to go to work.

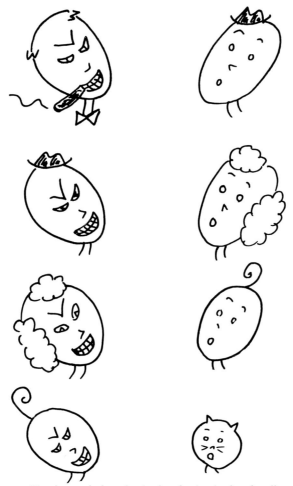

DISPLACEMENT: The boss rebukes the husband, the husband yells at the wife, the wife scolds the child and the child gets mad at the cat. The cat? Maybe he eats a mouse and in retaliation the mouse will probably give the cat a bellyache!

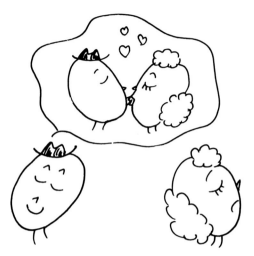

PROJECTION: In reality she dislikes him but he has projected his feelings of love to her, therefore he believes she loves him.

COMPENSATION: He compensates for his loss of hair early in life by wearing a toupee'.

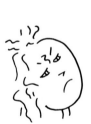 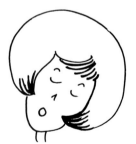

OVER-COMPENSATION: She would like very much to wear one of the puffy hair styles to hide her undersized head and thin hair but since she has neither the skill nor enough hair to do so, says she hates the new hair styles, they are ridiculous and she would not be caught dead in one.

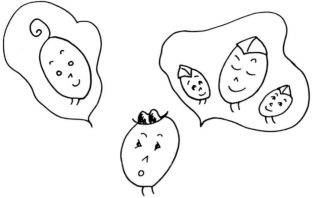

SUBLIMATION: He strongly desires a son but he is sterile so he becomes a Scout leader and has many 'sons.'

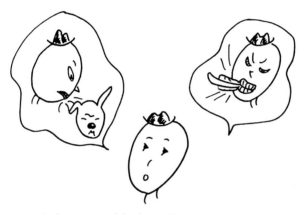

SUBSTITUTION: A dog runs and barks at him and he feels a strong urge to bite it but knows that such behavior would be unacceptable. Later when he buys a hot dog he unconsciously bites it viciously while eating it thereby releasing his tension.

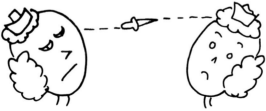

RATIONALIZATION: She played around on her days off and didn't get her cap ironed so she tells her supervisor (and herself) that she was too ill to get it done and everyone is just lucky that she even made it to work.

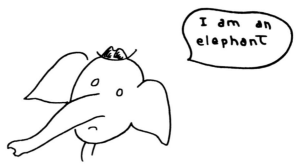

CONDENSATION: He is obese, has a large nose and outsize ears. He always performs at parties when asked and is secretly afraid of mice. So when he says 'I am an elephant' he is really saying all these things about himself.

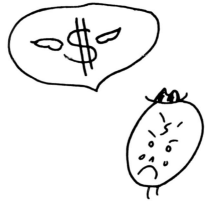

SYMBOLISM: A dollar sign is the symbol of all his unhappiness and every time he sees one he has a fit of weeping because it reminds him that he lost his fortune in 1929. (Wife too!)

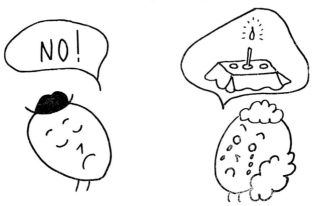

REGRESSION: She wants to go out to dinner, hubby says NO. To get her way she regresses to that point in her childhood when tears promptly got her what she wanted.

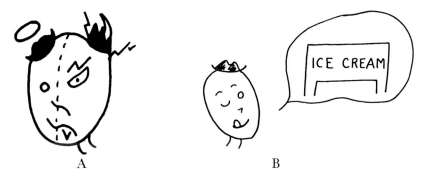

A. DISSOCIATION: This fellow has two selves—good and bad. He's a 'good' guy most of the time and works in a bank where there is great pressure from his superiors. He occasionally becomes the 'bad' guy and burglarizes stores. He has no recollection of his 'bad' self when he is 'good' and vice versa. His 'bad' activities unconsciously release his tension suffered at work.

B. COMPULSION: In order to feel comfortable he must lick his lips and wink his eye each time he passes an ice cream sign.

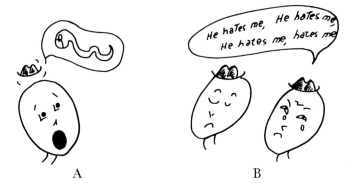

A. PHOBIA: He has become abnormally afraid of infestation by worms (vermiphobia).

B. OBSESSION: His friend became slightly miffed one day but he has become obsessed with the idea that his friend hates him.

symptoms of mental illness that send a person to a mental hospital, but it is the fact that the people around him can no longer stand his behavior. Early detection of these disturbances in an individual's personality will aid in correcting the situation before hospitalization becomes necessary.

When these behavioral patterns are used to excess and become inadequate in assisting the individual in reaching a solution to his pain and conflict, he begins to pile defense upon defense, thus leading to the production of symptoms which in turn cause his frame of reference to become more and more unrealistic.

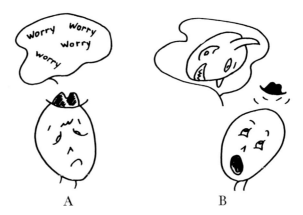

A. ANXIETY: The individual suffers in a state of apprehension, pain and fear, the reason unapparent. It is a reaction to the threat of a loss.

B. HALLUCINATION: The individual has a false perception; it can be tactile, auditory, olfactory or visual.

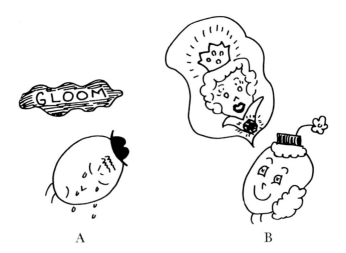

A. DEPRESSION: The individual suffers an inconsolable grief with feelings the reason for which is buried in the unconscious. Is a reaction to a loss.

B. DELUSION: The individual has a false belief, usually being one which is exactly the opposite of reality such as poverty versus status, power and wealth.

Chapter X

CLASSIFICATION AND DESCRIPTION OF
MENTAL ILLNESSES

INTRODUCTION

THE assignment of names of mental illnesses to an outline in a book is fairly easy to do. The method most commonly used is to group the types of illnesses by the kinds of symptoms which are characteristic of each. Every profession has its own jargon and the entire field of psychiatry, and psychiatric nursing, certainly has its own. However, psychiatry has come a long way since some of the words were coined and the words no longer mean what they once did. For example, "demented" and "dementia" used to mean literally the loss of one's mind. We have gradually come to realize that these terms were misleading; that a person didn't "lose" his mind. Many times the psychiatric "labeling" of a patient can produce untold harm. But until the profession as a whole accepts other methods of describing mental illnesses, the established labels will continue to be used.

One of the first things which you will learn about mental illnesses is that no matter how many patients there are on a ward, grouped under one classification, no *two* patients will exhibit exactly the *same* symptoms.

Mental illnesses are usually divided into two major categories, the psychoses and the psychoneuroses. In addition, there is a large group of disturbances which are classed as "Personality Disorders." Simplified versions of the various classifications are given in the following paragraphs.

THE PSYCHONEUROSES

The disturbances grouped under this heading usually refer to those of the emotional make-up of the individual rather than of the mind itself. The psychoneurotic patient, if admitted to a State hospital, does not as a rule remain in residence for any great period of time. The individual does not lose contact with reality (life as it is). The chief symptom of these disorders is "anxiety". The way in which the person attempts to handle this anxiety results in the symptoms of the various specific types.

Anxiety State, or Anxiety Reaction

This occurs in people who are the worrying type. They always seem tense physically as well as emotionally. They seem to be in constant fear that something unpleasant is going to happen, although what it is they cannot say. Many times when you say that you are "afraid that something will happen if I don't do so and so . . .", in reality you are "anxious".

A certain amount of tension is normal, it being the form in which both our mind and our body responds to a situation which demands increased effort. If we had no tension at all we could not adequately handle the demands which life makes on us. The person who is relatively normal will develop a temporary increase in tension under circumstances of physical or psychological stress. After the demanding situation has subsided, the tension usually eases off. If a person is under stress for an unusually long period of time, or if he has the sort of temperament which over reacts to stress, he may develop a number of physical symptoms associated with tension. They may be symptoms of a physical nature such as a headache, stiffness in the back of the neck, gastrointestional cramps and insomnia. Emotional symptoms such as restlessness and irritability may also occur.

Fear and *anxiety* are two emotional responses related to tension. Fear is often called forth by real physical danger and the body responds with a realistic response in which it prepares to do something about the danger. In the case of anxiety, the individual is responding not to an actual physical danger but to an intangible and often unidentified feeling of being threatened. Since there is no appropriate physical outlet for this feeling, the tension builds up instead of being discharged, and the person may become distraught, highly agitated, hysterical or immobilized. The fact that anxiety is often based upon nonphysical threats does not mean that it is necessarily unrealistic. In fact, it tends to occur at certain periods in a person's life when he is undergoing changes either in his own development or in his life situations. At these critical points in life, either new demands are being made upon the individual or his customary sources of security are being threatened. *Anxiety* is characteristic of adolescence, during the early years of marriage, during the initial experience of parenthood, during job changes and in old age.

Depressive Reaction

This condition may be masked or "covered up" by the physical complaints which the patient describes to you, such as "I'm tired, exhausted, my family is too much for me; I wake up in the middle of the night and can't go back to sleep." You would not know that the patient was depressed if he did not state that he was; however, the reason he gives is an excuse, not the real cause. It is usually due to the person's inability to accept or adapt themselves to some happening which for the time being destroyed their sense of security or has made them feel frustrated and useless.

Phobic Reaction

The individuals who are prone to suffer from various fears are emotionally related to those who suffer from anxiety. A "phobia" is fixed on a particular worry or fear, however, such as of being shut in a closed space, or of heights or as to the state of one's health. If a person is overly concerned about his health, he is called a "hypochondriac" and is suffering from "hypochondria." Many times the individual seems to be "enjoying poor health."

Obsessive-compulsive Reaction

The symptoms of this disorder are the result of unwanted ideas which occur over and over again in the person's mind, associated with an unwanted urge to perform an act or ritual. The individual may regard his ideas and actions as being unreasonable but in spite of this, is compelled to carry out his rituals. An example of a mild form is that of the man who must step over every crack in the sidewalk while on his way to work.

Conversion Reaction (also known as hysterical reaction)

This condition occurs in both sexes and at all ages, but it is more common among females. The condition was originally thought to be caused by the wandering of the womb within the body. These patients are people who as a rule are very imaginative and tend to dramatize everything that happens to them. The emotional disturbance may result in a variety of conditions some of which are loss of voice for speaking, loss of memory, loss of sensation in certain areas of the body, inability to walk or inability to use an arm or hand.

Depressive Reaction

In this disorder, the person relieves to a degree his anxiety by withdrawing into a mood of depression and belittling of himself. This type of depression is of a much milder degree than that of a psychotic depression.

THE PSYCHOSES

These disorders are the result of severe emotional disturbances which have disrupted the normal manner of thinking, feeling and acting of a person to such a degree that he can no longer do his work or get along socially. The disorders are usually divided into two headings, the *organic* and the *functional,* each in turn being subdivided.

I. Organic Psychoses

These disturbances each have some specific physical condition which produces symptoms of abnormal behavior. They may be associated with:

1. *Toxins,* or poisons from either within the body or from outside the body.
   a. Infection from disease, an example being syphilis, can cause mental illness.
   b. Drugs such as the bromides.
   c. Poisons such as from lead.
2. Intoxication, as from alcohol.
   a. Delirium tremens is an example.

3. Trauma, or injury to the head and brain.
4. Tumors in the brain.
5. Convulsive disorders.
6. Cerebral arteriosclerosis, or "hardening of the arteries" in the brain.
7. Other circulatory disturbances.
8. Other disturbances of growth, nutrition or metabolism.

II. Functional Psychoses

These disturbances have no physical reason for an explanation of the individual's strange behavior.

1. Involutional Depression

Also known as "involutional psychotic reaction" and "involutional melancholia." This condition tends to develop in the late forties and early fifties in both male and female.

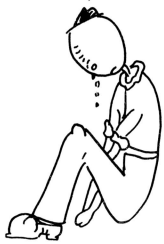

It usually coincides with the menopause, or "change of life" in women. Its outstanding symptom is one of depression.

2. Manic-depressive Psychoses

Also known as "manic-depressive reactions," "affective reactions," "cyclothymia." Symptoms may first appear

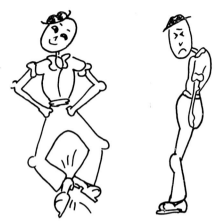

during the teen years but usually appear during the twenties or later. Individual's behavior is characterized by mood swings.

3.   *Paranoid Psychoses*

Also known as "paranoid reactions" and "paranoid states." Individual's behavior is characterized by suspicion and distrust. The condition known as "Paranoia" is characterized by a gradually developing, complicated set of delusions which may serve to endow the patient with superior ability, power or position. In general, the rest of the person's personality is unchanged. As a rule these people are not in state hospitals.

4.   *Schizophrenia*

Also known as "dementia praecox," and "schizophrenic reactions." Four types are generally described: the simple, the hebephrenic, the catatonic and the paranoid. As a whole this group accounts for about one half of all the patients in mental hospitals and about one quarter of all hospital patients in the U.S. About 125,000 new patients with this condition are admitted to mental hospitals each year. Their behavior is characterized by an apparent indifference to everything and everyone about them. They live in a "dream world" which is more satisfactory to them than any effort to face reality. They are not interested in their personal appearance and it is difficult to get their attention. They have a language all their own. He may smile frequently as though in response to voices or he may be mute and unresponsive to all external stimuli.

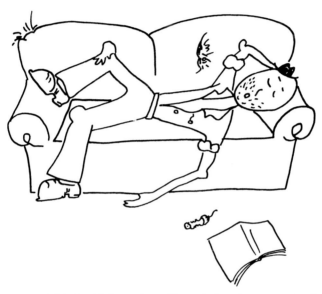

SIMPLE: The individual withdraws from life and doesn't care or try to achieve.

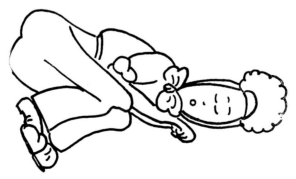

HEBEPHRENIA: The individual experiences complete withdrawal and decompensation, extensive regression and personality disintegration with delusions, hallucinations and infantile behavior.

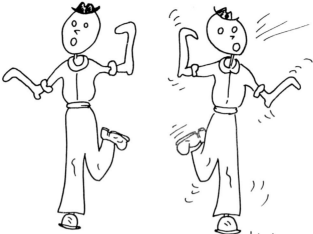

CATATONIC: The individual alternates between periods of stupor with odd postures and stereotyping and periods of intense excited activity.

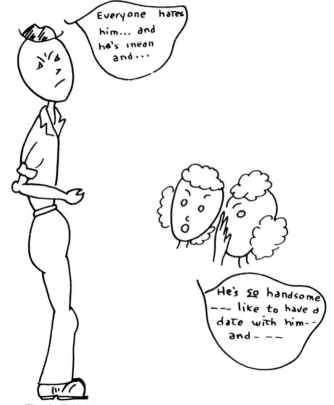

PARANOID: The individual shows no evidence of serious personality disorganization other than a well-developed and intricate system of delusions usually of persecution, although sometimes these delusions are ones of grandeur.

PERSONALITY DISORDERS

The individual in this group seems to suffer very little from anxiety and show very little reaction to stress. The disorder is diagnosed by the life-long pattern of behavior or action rather than by mental or emotional symptoms.

1. The inadequate personality.
2. Schizoid personality.
3. Cyclothymic personality.
4. Paranoid personality.

The *sociopathic personality* is also known as the "constitutional psychopathic state" or "psychopathic personality."

The common types are usually given as reactions, antisocial or dysocial; or with sexual deviation, or with addiction, either alcohol or drug.

The outstanding feature of all these types is their inability to benefit from experience. They seem to be "at war" with society, everybody and everything in it. Regardless of how much they may be criticized or may be punished, their acts will be repeated time after time.

Chapter XI

METHODS USED IN TREATING THE
MENTALLY ILL

INTRODUCTION

The ways and means of treating the mentally ill individual are varied, some being simple and clearly defined; others, more devious and mysterious. The techniques may be adapted to meet treatment needs of either the mentally ill or the mentally retarded, depending upon the physician and the hospital in which he practices. The methods may be grouped under three categories:

1. Somatic, or physical agents used on the body.
2. Social therapy.
3. Psychotherapy, or treatment of the mind.

Bear in mind that this grouping is academic, that when you are personally caring for patients, the *total* person as related to his *total* environment must be taken into consideration.

SOMATIC THERAPIES

The somatic therapies range from hydrotherapy which has been used since ancient times to the latest "tranquilizer" which may be introduced on the market tomorrow.

Hydrotherapy, or Treatment by Water

The two procedures most commonly used are the continuous tub bath and the wet sheet pack, each being ordered for the purpose of reducing anxiety, tension and overactivity. The exact procedures for their application will vary somewhat among hospitals. Neither treatment should ever be given without a doctor's order. One of the

162

most important parts of either treatment is the attitude of the psychiatric technician who administers, or assists with, the treatment. An
explanation of the treatment should always be given the patient even
though he may appear to be so disturbed that he doesn't understand
what is happening. Unfortunately, the wet sheet pack has been mis-
used many times in that the patient is given the impression that he
is being "packed" for punishment. It should not be necessary to re-
mind you that no treatment should be given a patient with the
thought of "punishing" him.

Insulin Shock, or Insulin Coma

Certain types of schizophrenic patients respond best to this
treatment. If the patient's illness is of six months or less duration the
results of treatment will be much better. In general, the older the
patient and the more chronic he has become the less the chances
are for improvement. The patient is given an injection of insulin
which may range from 10 units to 200 or more units. This causes
the sugar content of the patient's blood to decrease to the degree
which causes a hypoglycemic, or insulin coma (or unconsciousness.)
The patient is usually permitted to remain in the coma stage for
about one hour after which he is revived by being given a glucose
(sugar) solution. This is done by a tube through the nose and into
the stomach or by intravenous injection. A full course of treatment
will usually consist of about fifty hours of coma; the number of
periods of coma and the degree of coma depending upon the
physician. Insulin therapy is expensive in that it requires considerable time plus a high ratio of trained personnel.

A modified form of insulin therapy in which smaller doses of
insulin are given the patients, can be handled with fewer personnel,
as the patients do not go into coma.

Electric Shock or Electro-convulsive Therapy

This treatment is especially effective for patients suffering from
depressions. At times it almost appears miraculous in its effect upon
an individual in the depression of involutional melancholia.

The actual procedure may vary slightly from hospital to hospital but in general it will consist of placing the patient on a hard

surface, a gag is inserted between his teeth and electrodes are applied to his temple areas by the use of a saline substance which will aid in conducting the electric current. Then a very carefully controlled electric current is passed through the patient's brain, which causes him to have a convulsion, which is very like an epileptic seizure. Electroshock is much less expensive than insulin therapy in that it is quicker, the average treatment requiring about three minutes, and does not require as many personnel. The treatment can be modified so that the convulsion will not be so severe, and elderly, or even infirm, patients can be given E.C.T.

Most authorities have stated that the "shock" therapies make patients more accessible to psychotherapy, or more "reachable" by others. This in turn leads to better socializing with others on the ward, as well as a greater willingness to participate in the various occupational and recreational activities provided by the hospital. The psychiatric technician on the treatment wards play a very important role in helping these patients concentrate on healthy activities, both physical and mental, and discouraging any tendency upon the part of the patient to brood, about their symptoms. The technician's attitude should be one of optimism and to be an understanding and sympathetic partner in encouraging the patients to take part in activities. Because patients who undergo electroshock usually have a period of confusion and loss of memory, they will need sincere reassurance that their amnesia, or memory loss, is only a temporary thing. After all, it can be a pretty frightening thing to think that you have forgotten everything you ever knew! In any discussion with the patient about his treatment it is wise to avoid the use of the words "electric" or "electro" shock. Many patients are frightened by the electrodes used and then they additionally hear the words "electric-shock" they are convinced that they are about to be electrocuted, with the resulting reaction being far from therapeutic.

Psychosurgery

This term refers to any surgical procedure used in treating mental disorders. Prefrontal lobotomy is the procedure most commonly referred to, it being a procedure in which a hole is made in the front part of the skull and certain parts of the nerve tracts in the frontal lobes of the brain are cut. Most authorities have agreed that it is a method of treatment which is to be used after all other therapies have proven to be of no avail. The drastic surgical procedures have not been used so much since the use of tranquilizing drugs has been so effective. Patients who have had lobotomies require a habit-training program which is similar to that planned for a mentally retarded child, because the patient has been surgically "reduced" to the level of a child. The psychiatric technician must possess an unlimited amount of patience in teaching these patients and will need to draw upon their imagination and initiative to keep the patients busy and occupied.

Narcotherapy (also known as narcoanalysis or as narcosynthesis)

This method of treatment consists of the use of sedative drugs to produce a drowsy, relaxed state on the part of the patient, during which the doctor questions the patient about his problems. Two of the drugs which are used are sodium amytal and sodium pentothal. These are the drugs which are commonly spoken of as "truth serum," but if an individual does not want to "tell all," no amount of drug will induce him to talk.

Fever Therapy

This method is used to treat general paresis, a condition caused by the infection of the brain and nerve tissue with syphilis. The fever is produced either by inoculating the patient with malaria or by the use of a specially constructed heat cabinet. The number of hours of high fever (over $103°F$) is prescribed by the doctor. The physical condition of the patient must also be carefully considered. Fever therapy may be preceded by treatment with arsenical drugs such as salvarsan or tryparsamide. In many cases the drugs are used following a course of fever treatments. However, these older methods of treating syphilis of all types have been nearly discontinued in favor of penicillin and other antibiotics. Large doses of penicillin carries very little risk to the patient, is rapid and is not as uncomfortable as fever treatments. A course of penicillin treatments may be repeated if the first course does not achieve the desired effects.

SOCIAL THERAPY

The physical act of being removed from a stressful situation and being admitted to a hospital is a form of treatment. However, in many institutions, starting with the admission procedure and continuing throughout the patient's progress through a series of wards, rigid hospital rules and regulations do very little to encourage a patient to have a sense of responsibility for themselves physically or socially. In recent years there has been a renewed interest in the use of the social environment as a positive means of treatment. More recognition has been given to the fact that patients can not only help themselves to a greater degree, if given the chance, but that they can also help their fellow patients, in some instances more so than the hospital staff. Exploration of more effective use of social treatments includes patient participation in plans for his therapy, patient self government, remotivation, group therapy and the "open door" for more wards. Home care programs, day or night care centers, and mental hygiene clinics have all helped to create a more positive social relationship between the hospital and the community. All of these concepts have positive expectations for the patient's improvement and eliminates the mental image of the psychiatric technician as the "guard who carries the keys."

In most state institutions there has always been the problem of over crowding with patients and understaffing with personnel, resulting over the years in the accumulation of many patients who received little more than custodial treatment. Many patients withdrew from life to the extent that they had forgotten how to talk and had lost all interest in the world and everything in it. A method which can be used by the psychiatric technician to "reach" this group of patients in a constructive and meaningful way is by the technique of remotivation. It is not psychotherapy in the strict sense of the word but is a simple method which the psychiatric technician can use to develop a group interaction with his patients. It can be adapted to any ward in the average mental institution and is especially helpful in establishing contact with the withdrawn, regressed, "chronic" patient. The technique of remotivation is based on five essential steps: (1) the climate of acceptance; (2) a bridge to reality; (3) sharing the world we live in; (4) an appreciation of the work of the world, and (5) the climate of appreciation. For more detailed information see Appendix D. As with any other treatment program, this would require the ward doctor's order for initiation.

DRUG THERAPY

Many drugs have been used in the treatment of mental illness through the years. Starting in 1953 in the United States, two types of drugs have been used with dramatic effect in the treatment of patients whose behavior was hyperactive, combative, angry or otherwise unapproachable. These same drugs and/or combination of drugs have been equally effective in the treatment of patients who for many years have been considered "chronic cases" and all but forgotten by society.

The drug treatment of mentally retarded patients has worked wonders in aiding in controlling such behavior as hyperactivity, assaultiveness, destructiveness, feeding problems and related problems. The drugs also aid in easing the anxieties, tensions and fears which tend to afflict the mentally retarded as well as the mentally ill.

These drugs fall into two categories, tranquilizers and energizers.

The tranquilizing agents can:

"(1) Enable the patient to make a more rapid, and more satisfactory adjustment to the hospital routine.

(2) Create a quieter, pleasanter and more orderly atmosphere that is, in itself, a source of comfort to the patients and an inspiration to the staff.

(3) Increase the patient's capacity to respond to other forms of treatment designed to speed his return to society.

(4) Promote greater sociability and better participation in ward activities.

(5) Improve appetite and eating habits.

(6) Promote better sleeping habits and lessen the frequency of nocturnal disturbances.

(7) Heighten patient interest in personal appearance and grooming.

(8) Reduce the number of injuries due to patients assaulting themselves, other patients or members of the staff.

(9) Help to prevent the destruction of clothing, furniture, bedding, etc., thereby lowering repair and replacement costs.

"Although the drugs are instrumental in controlling the patient's symptoms, there are many things they *cannot* do. They cannot substitute for other psychiatric techniques, adequate facilities and dedicated, knowledgeable personnel. Their usefulness lies in the fact that they often help to bring the patient within reach of those who seek to help him, and thereby permit the initiation of more advanced treatment programs." *

"Ataraxics" is another term used for the tranquilizer group of drugs, the term coming from a Greek word which means peace of mind and lack of confusion. Some of the better known drug names are:

Reserpine (trade name Serpasil®)

This produces a mild sedative effect, and results in a sense of well-being associated with lessening of tension and a calm, relaxed behavior on the part of the patient. It lowers the blood pressure more than any of the other tranquilizers.

Meprobamate (trade name Miltown® and Equanil®)

This drug has proven particularly effective in relieving such conditions as tension headaches, sleeplessness, and tensions associated with the menstrual period.

Frenquel

This drug has been used to relieve the acute confusion found in some schizophrenic disorders and for some senile patients who become confused.

---

*Smith Kline and French Laboratories: *Psychiatric Nurse's Guide to SK&F Tranquilizing Drugs.* 1500 Spring Garden St., Philadelphia, 1964, p. 4.

Chlorpromazine (trade name Thorazine®)

This is one of the most widely used of tranquilizers. Regardless of the diagnosis of the patient, it will calm them all, with very few exceptions. Patients who are combative, overactive, excited, noisy, anxious or confused will become more accessible for other therapies and activities. Occasionally undesirable effects such as jaundice and liver involvement, or lowered blood pressure occur, but they clear up if the drug is discontinued. *Pacatal®, Sparine®, Compazine®* and *Trilafon®* are some of the other more commonly prescribed tranquilizing agents.

The group of drugs which are known as *Energizers* are used to treat various states of depression as well as to overcome the drowziness and fatigue which sometimes follows the use of the tranquilizers. Among such drugs which have been used successfully are *Ritalin®, Meratran®* and *Marsalid®*.

No pill, however, will take the place of skillfully directed human relationships in restoring the mentally ill to health. No pill can substitute for a wholesome environment, training, or schooling for the mentally retarded. Although some of the drugs seem to have a favorable influence on the patients' ability to learn, the drugs do not increase the actual intelligence quotient. The fact that the I.Q. scores for individual patients have improved, most investigators believe that the improvement is due to the drugs' effects on secondary symptoms rather than the mental deficiency itself. An example would be that of a hyperactive, distractable child whose attention could never be focused on a learning situation but as a result of the use of a tranquilizer, the child could be taught to concentrate even though it might be for a few minutes at a time to start with. The use of such drugs aid in making patients more accessible to all therapeutic methods, especially in the area of the interpersonal relationships which are so essential in psychiatric nursing.

You must also keep in mind the fact that these drugs do not cure mental illnesses; they have just made the symptoms easier for everyone to live with including the patient. The psychiatric technician must encourage and assist the patient to help himself to adjust to his environment. Because more patients have become more cooperative as a result of the tranquilizers, the routines of both patients and psychiatric technicians have become more active and meaningful. There is greater need for the services of the occupational, recreational, industrial, educational and musical therapies, and in many institutions the psychiatric technician will be the "right hand man" acting for these therapists at ward level.

GROUP THERAPY WITH THE MENTALLY ILL

Many patients have withdrawn from life to the extent that they have forgotten how to talk and have lost all interest in the world and everything in it. A method which the psychiatric technician can use to reach this group of patients in a constructive and meaningful way is by remotivation. It can be adopted to any ward in the average mental institution and is especially helpful in establishing contact with the withdrawn, regressed, chronic and/or the elderly patients.

Social environment can be used as a positive means of treatment. In recent years more recognition has been given to the fact that patients can not only help themselves to a greater degree, if given the chance, but that they can also help their fellow patients, in some instances more so than the hospital staff. Exploration of more effective use of social treatments includes patient participation in plans for his therapy, patient self-government, remotivation, group therapy and the "open-door" for more wards.

Various methods of group therapy are instruments which the therapist uses to assist in the therapeutic process. Psychotherapy is basically the process by which the therapist shares an experience with his patient. Whether the therapist calls himself a psychiatrist, psychoanalyst, psychologist, psychiatric nurse, a psychiatric technician, or a rehabilitation therapist, the psychotherapy he performs is primarily the process of sharing an experience with the patient. Psychotherapy should be a twenty-four-hour-a-day-operation and the psychiatric technician especially should utilize group therapy methods only as an aid in the matter of sharing an experience with his patients.

Two methods of group therapy which psychiatric technician personnel can conduct, with beneficial results for the patients, are:

    1. Those designed for the purpose of helping the patient to communicate.

2. Those planned to assist the patient to adjust to the group.

Neither method is in any way analytical; they are for the specific purpose of bringing the patient back to reality. The patient is offered a non-threatening situation in which he is able to respond normally "right now."

No patient is scheduled for any type of therapy without a physician's order.

The sessions should not be scheduled more than once a day nor more than five times per week.

MOTIVATIONAL GROUP THERAPY

Definition

A method of group bibliotherapy (reading) designed for operation by psychiatric technician personnel in the treatment of patients who are unable to properly handle verbal communication.

Very little equipment is needed:

1. Seating facilities for patients and therapists.
2. For each patient and therapist a printed copy of the material to be read.
3. A watch or clock to check time.

Suggested seating plan:

```
    o o o o o o o           o—patient
@ o o o o o o o @           @—therapist
    o o o o o o o
          @
```

Ideal ratio is seven patients to each therapist.
21 patients and 3 therapists is an ideal group.
Total number of patients participating should never exceed 35

Reading material should be:

A factual story without dialogue. The story should be typed or printed on single standard typewriter size sheets and the sentences arranged in numbered sequence. Material from grade school or high school history books is probably the best source of this kind of reading matter.

Following is an example of reading material that may be used:

Gold Discovery in California

1. Gold was discovered near Sacramento, California, in the year of 1849 by Captain Sutter.
2. News of the discovery spread like wildfire and within a few months people were flocking to California.
3. Villages and towns soon appeared in all areas where there was a possibility of finding gold.
4. Many people came to California on covered wagons and a large number arrived by sail-boat.
5. Covered wagons usually traveled over the now famous "Overland Trail" and the sail-boats journeyed around South America.
6. Etc., etc. . . . .

Method of Operation

The lead therapist reads sentence #1 and then selects a patient to read sentence #2. This operation represents a cycle. After this cycle has been repeated several times, the lead therapist changes places with one of the assistant therapists. The lead therapist directs the session and the assistant therapist gives help to patients when they are selected for reading.

It is important that the therapists not stimulate patients to discuss the material being read. The goal of this method of group therapy is to help the patient to read. When he is ready to discuss material, he is qualified for advancement to one of the other methods of group therapy where discussion is the instrument of therapy.

The Lead Therapist

The lead therapist is stationed at the head of the group. He is the director of the group session in operation. He selects which patient is to read and decides when one of the assistant therapists is to take his place.

The Assistant Therapist

Assistant therapists station themselves with the patient group. When a patient is asked to read, the assistant therapist nearest the patient goes to his side and gives whatever help is needed. The assistant therapist takes the place of the lead therapist when so ordered by the lead therapist.

Patients who find it difficult to talk are, to a great degree, unable to think of words to use. In this method of therapy, we more or less "put words in their mouths" by providing reading material. Often, when operating this method of group therapy, patients unable to utter a single word will say several words as they read their assigned sentence. After repeated sessions of reading the patient learns that words can flow from his mouth without ill effects to himself. Hence, he is given a chance to overcome his symptom of "blocked speech" in a group situation that is non-threatening to any of the participants.

Once a patient is capable of handling "words put in his mouth" he is ready for the next level of group therapy which utilizes a method whereby "he selects for himself the words that come from his mouth."

In a situation where there is a shortage of unit personnel, a patient audience may be added to the regular method. Patients are then classified as the participants and audience. The participants carry on the regular session while the audience merely observes the operation.

REORIENTATION GROUP THERAPY

Definition

A method of group therapy designed for use by psychiatric technician personnel in the treatment of patients having difficulty with simple thinking and spontaneous speech.

Equipment needed and suggested seating plan:

1. Seating facilities for patients and therapist.
2. Reading material for the therapist to use.
3. A watch or clock for checking the time.

Suggested seating plan:

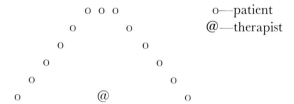

The ideal ratio is 14 patients to each therapist. Less than seven patients per therapist lowers the efficiency of the session.

Type of reading material to use:

A factual story, such as an article from a magazine, newspaper, or a portion from a history book, will provide excellent reading material. The therapist should be careful not to use stories that are closely associated with the life history of any participating patients. At each session new material should be used.

Method of Operation

1. The therapist, or one of his chosen patients, reads the selected story.
2. As various items appear in the reading, the therapist interrupts the reader and asks questions of the patients concerning the item.

The therapist should refrain from asking questions that require a statement of the patients opinion. Following is an example of the type of questions used by the therapist in this method of group therapy:

Suppose the subject matter being used concerns the history of gold discovery in California. The reading proceeds until the item "gold" appears. Here the therapist interrupts the reading and asks the question, "John Doe, have you ever owned anything gold?" "Jack Smith, in making jewelry, what substitute is used for gold?" Attention is invited to the fact that the questions asked above do not require the patient to state his concepts or opinions. With experience, the therapist will develop the ability to think of suitable questions with ease. The saying, "practice makes perfect" applies well to this situation.

In the broadest sense, there are two types of thinking, which can be called "simple thinking" and "conceptual thinking." The meaning which an individual places on information which he receives represents his opinion, or concept, of the situation in question. Response to perceptions which are not conditioned by one's opinion may be considered to be "simple thinking." (It is impossible for anyone to accomplish a pure form of "simple thinking," however, it is a term which can be used to aid in establishing a basis for understanding therapy objectives.)

It is a fact that mentally ill people behave the way they do because their "conceptual thinking apparatus" is not operating well. The concept many patients have of themselves and you, and of their environment in general, is not correct and in conformity with the rules of culture. The patient is, therefore, more likely to give an intelligent answer when asked a question that does not require "conceptual thinking" than when he is asked a question which demands his opinion.

The first step to be taken in the process of giving therapy to a patient who is withdrawn and mentally confused, is to help him accomplish "simple thinking." Reorientation Group Therapy is designed specifically for this purpose.

DISCUSSION GROUP THERAPY

This is a group therapy method which can also be carried out by psychiatric technician personnel in the treatment of patients needing exercise in participating as members of a discussion group.

The ideal ratio is seven patients to each therapist. Not more than 14 patients per therapist should be used.

Materials which can be used for discussion include:
1. Newspaper or magazine article.
2. Factual material from books.
3. Radio or television program.
4. Moving picture program.
5. Observation or participation in an event.

Method of Operation

The session is divided into two parts: (1) the preparation period, and (2) the discussion period.

The Preparation Period

During this period the group membership is given material to be discussed. If the subject matter is from a book or newspaper, the therapist or a chosen patient reads to the group. Should the therapist decide that the discussion material will be a radio or television program, he arranges for the group to obtain such information. Whatever the source of material, the therapist will schedule his group to secure that information.

The Discussion Period

During this period the group, with the help of the therapist discusses the material it has gathered during the preparation period. The therapist, while assuming an attitude of observer, steers the course of discussion.

Each discussion should consider these phases of deliberation: (1) the motive; (2) the goal, and (3) factors regarding attainment of the goal. The period of discussion should last for not more than an hour, with a five or ten minute rest period at the midway point.

In most cases, it might be advisable for the therapist to first review the material to be discussed. At the termination of the discussion, a recapitulation of what has been said is a good procedure to follow.

Chapter XII

THE ROLE OF NURSING PERSONNEL*

INTRODUCTION

THE mentally ill person has in the past always been looked upon as a threat to society, therefore to be removed from society. The asylum provided for the individual, gave custodial care, where the peculiarities of the mentally ill met a reasonable degree of acceptance and where nursing personnel gave basic nursing care.

A mentally ill person, due to the nature of his illness, is unable to assess his own needs. He may, for example, feel the desire to die, may wish to starve, or to avoid contact with anyone, all of which are symptoms of his illness. Psychiatric nursing personnel must learn to recognize and evaluate the patient's needs.

As the result of long experience, education and research, it has been determined by many authorities that the needs of mentally ill patients have been misunderstood and the type of nursing care provided had many disadvantages. The removal of responsibility and the refraining from judgment and criticism of patients' behavior led to a loss of self-respect and dignity, as well as an acceptance by patients and staff of living standards incompatible with recovery and zest for life. It led to the development of an "institutionalization syndrome."

The most important aspect of current thinking is an awareness of the social interaction which takes place between patients and the community in which they live. We no longer see the patients' needs

*Refers to any person: Registered nurse, psychiatric technician, licensed vocational nurse, hospital aide, ward attendant and related titles, who are most closely associated with and care and provide for those who are either mentally and/or physically ill.

solely as those of a sick person who passively submits to the care of the staff. Instead, we understand that the patient, as a member of society, affects by his illness all the people with whom he has any relationships, and in turn is affected by the community, be it the hospital, the family, his work situation or the community as a whole. The patient's illness, whatever its cause, manifests itself in his relationships with people. Recovery and rehabilitation must take place in the patient's social setting. The patient's needs have many facets, such as:

1. Requiring some technical nursing such as that related to bathing, feeding, dressing and administration of medications.
2. A need for therapeutic personal relationships with trained members of the staff, i.e., the doctors, nurses and other psychiatric nursing personnel, which enable the patient to work through his emotional difficulties and to accept the other phases of treatment. Such relationships can be developed in an atmosphere of a therapeutic community.
3. A need for social relationships and for the opportunity to relearn and practice social interaction. The latter is especially true for the patient who through long hospitalization has lost all contact with society.

The psychiatric technician, as well as other members of the treatment team, learns to make use of basic nursing procedures as a medium through which emotional contacts can be made. During his period of illness the patient may look upon the nursing person as a mother, or as a protector, or as a figure of authority.

Interpersonal skills interact and overlap with the technical skills and with the social skills which the psychiatric technician must bring to bear on the community in which the patient's treatment takes place. Because the social setting in which the patient is cared for affects his recovery, the nursing person must develop the ability to utilize the whole group for the treatment of each individual. She must understand the effect people have on each other, the way her own attitude affects her patients, what reactions the patients' behavior elicits from her and how staff morale or differences of opinions about patients' treatment find repercussions on the ward. There are many other factors which must also be learned, such as:

1. The way people express themselves indirectly.
2. How to understand what an individual means when he is silent or when he covers his real feelings by small talk.
3. An understanding of relationships between the patient and his family, the family's way of expressing feelings of guilt or anxiety, as well as trying to understand the family's difficulties as well as the patients'.

The nursing of the mentally ill is a cooperative effort between the staff and the patient, in which the patient is as active as the psychiatric technician, the nurse or the doctor. The patient's treatment and rehabilitation take place in relation to communal living. The patient must be helped to find his place in society; the ward or hospital society at first, later his family circle and his own community. He must learn how to live an active life, how to assume responsibility for his own actions and to be concerned for others. He can learn this if he takes an active part in the running of the hospital and if he assumes an active role in his own treatment. The hospital can provide opportunities for patients to learn to achieve greater success in social situations by helping them to develop feelings of security with other people. Developing a warm, home-like, accepting ward atmosphere is one of the major therapeutic contributions which the psychiatric technician can make to improve the patient's hospital experience.

As we become aware of the patients' needs in relation to his environment, we realize that all the people in his environment in some way become involved in learning to recognize that the patient must be a partner in the plan for recovery and not be merely a passive recipient of care. Within the hospital all members of the team—doctors, nurses, psychiatric technicians, social workers, psychologists, rehabilitation therapists, teachers—must pool their skills and knowledge.

The acquisition of technical skills, that is, learning of specific nursing care procedures is relatively easy even though they may vary from ward to ward or from hospital to hospital. But learning to understand human relationships is a difficult task; it requires much experience in addition to the knowledge obtained from textbooks.

Your primary approach should be planned to reduce fear and

anxiety, promote self-confidence in the patient and a sense of affection while at the same time providing the necessary physical and emotional protection for the patient.

APPROACH TO THE PATIENT

There are certain general principles that apply to the care of patients, regardless of the behavior pattern exhibited by a particular type of mental illness. The first contact which you have with a patient is, hopefully, the beginning of a therapeutic relationship, this first contact being the all-important basis for all future communications between you and the patient.

An impairment in the ability to communicate effectively is one of the most outstanding symptoms of mental illness. Skillful communication is, therefore, one of the most important arts which you must learn in psychiatric nursing. The concept of communication should include all those processes by which people influence one another. The feeling of relief after successful communication molds people in such a way that they begin to seek the companionship of others.

Communication can be either verbal or non-verbal as well as a variety of combinations of both.

Talking is one way by which you let a patient know whether or not you accept him. It will not necessarily be the words of your conversation, but the tone of your voice and the expression on your face which will evoke responses from the patient. You may be verbalizing all the correct words using correct grammar and descriptive phrases, but a gesture, or even your posture, may unfortunately convey to the patient a feeling that he is being rejected by you.

The basic rule for talking with patients is the same as for any social conversation: be courteous and offer the patient ample opportunity to participate. When initiating a conversation with either one or a group of patients, it is well to start talking about some commonplace subject, such as the weather, which is not apt to stir up intense feelings. The main difference between social type conversation with patients and that with your friends is that you do not relate details of your personal life (such as the quarrel you may have had with your boy friend the night before), to patients. You should focus on the needs and interests of the patient, not on your own! Until you get to know the patient, it is a good idea to follow the patient's lead in selecting topics for conversation. In contrast to the social type of conversation which can be carried on with all patients, a therapeutic conversation is conducted with a selected individual or with a selected group. This is usually done in cooperation with the doctor and other members of the ward team. Unless you are given specific instructions to do otherwise, you should avoid giving a patient an interpretation of his behavior.

Even though you may "know all about your patients" *careless talk* can create unnecessary anxiety and even retard the therapeutic process for a patient. A patient's reaction will depend upon such factors as his specific illness, what he hears and how he interprets what he hears. (He may hear something that you didn't actually say!) Before speaking, pause and consider the effect your words may have on patients; sensitive areas which should be avoided include:

1. Insisting to a depressed patient that he be more cheerful.
2. Instructing an overactive patient to sit down and be quiet.
3. Direct contradiction of a patient's expression of psychotic ideas.
4. Urging a withdrawn patient to initiate and complete group activities.
5. Showing off your knowledge of medical and psychiatric terminology in front of patients.
6. Focusing attention on a patient's weaknesses.
7. Indifference, threats, or sharp commands.
8. Careless conversation where patients can over hear you.

Listening is also involved in communication. The role of being a "listener" cannot be over-emphasized. There are many people in our society who have never had anyone listen to what they have to say; if such an individual becomes emotionally ill, perhaps the most therapeutic thing that could happen to him would be to have a good listener. Perhaps you have had the experience, in a social setting, of having someone thank you for the wonderful evening that he has had with you (not with the group) and you reply with a wish that you could have been more vivacious. The pleasure which you had provided was in being a "listener" instead of a "talker"!

Being a good listener is one of the most difficult tasks which you will have to perform in psychiatric nursing. It is difficult because of two basic factors: traditional concepts of what constitutes nursing and your personal anxieties. Usually nursing personnel have been taught to keep busy in performing procedures or in "doing something for the patients." When you attempt being a "listener" there is nothing to be handled or manipulated and you have guilt feelings about doing nothing. Your anxiety about doing "nothing" is compounded if you become aware of fellow employees surreptitious remarks about you just "sitting around, with the patients, doing nothing." You will not become a skillful listener unless you are able to develop some means of handling your personal anxiety. You can be said to be on the way to becoming a good "listener" if you can concentrate on what is being said and the feeling that is being communicated, rather than on what you are going to say when the opportunity arises.

SHARING YOUR TIME

There are times when you need not talk or even appear to listen, but you just sit with a patient. There is no "fool proof" mode of behavior toward all your patients or even toward anyone at different times. Because the mentally ill do have the problem of communicating, your quiet presence says many things to many patients; the withdrawn patient who is desperately lonely may begin to trust you during such a time and to the hyperactive patient your sitting quietly may suggest to him that he do the same. Sitting by the side of a depressed patient doesn't require physical contact at all to provide the type of reassurance needed to make him feel wanted and worthwhile.

Sitting with a patient, or near by him, is one method of reassuring him that you are interested in him as a person and that he may be as sick as he needs to be. It is well to remember that patient behavior is changed by emotional experience, not by rational explanation, and that if a patient could be *reasoned* out of his psychiatric ideas and behavior he would not need treatment in a hospital.

In psychiatric nursing, you must listen with the heart as well as with the mind and be prepared to give, with the expectation of no return other than the happiness of seeing patients get well.

CARE OF THE SCHIZOPHRENIC, OR THE WITHDRAWN, PREOCCUPIED PATIENT

Patients with a diagnosis of some type of schizophrenia occupy about one half of the mental hospital beds in the U.S. Many have grown old on a "backward" or on a "continued treatment ward." As a group the individuals who develop schizophrenic behavior are those who have a great deal of trouble in establishing relationships with other people. They seem to never have had a feeling of warmth for their fellow man and are prone to withdraw from human contact. The disease may develop at any age, the onset being slow, but it is first noticed during adolescence and the early twenties. The person becomes preoccupied with his day dreams, to the exclusion of all interest in daily living. He may become sullen and suspicious, or may go through a series of posturing, or may have outbreaks of silly laughter, or may have unexpected spells of violence. His response to anyone who extends offers of assistance is met with indifference.

With very few exceptions, schizophrenic patients will have a lifelong history of unhappiness in his emotional adjustments to life. His childhood has been an unhappy one, having been made to feel extremely insecure during the most helpless time in his life bcause of the conflict and anxieties of his parents or others who cared for him. Personality disturbances may be noted quite early in the life of a child and measures can be taken to overcome the problem.

DEVELOPMENT OF EMOTIONAL PROBLEMS IN CHILDHOOD

The child's symptoms may be of a neurotic type, a relatively mild type of behavior, or the behavior can be so strange and queer that it will be diagnosed as psychotic, it usually being a childhood schizophrenia.

The subject of childhood psychosis or schizophrenia, or infantile autism as many prefer to call it, is a condition which is still unfamiliar to us. *Autism* was first identified in 1943 and is presently regarded by most pediatricians and child psychiatrists as the earliest appearing and most severe problem of emotional illness in very young children. Autism was, and is, frequently mistaken for mental retardation which it resembles, and until recently most of these children were placed in state institutions as "mentally deficient." General retardation may become, in time, the primary characteristic of the child's disturbance if he goes untreated.

It is important that doctors, nurses and others involved in care of children become acquainted with the early signs of the condition because a "wait and see" attitude delays the initiation of the early therapy which is so necessary if the child is to be successfully treated. The earliest signs of autistic behavior is most difficult to describe in clear-cut terms. A sudden change in the child's disposition and appearance as a result of such events as a separation from the parents or the birth of a sibling, is most easily recognized by the parents. A more insidious onset may be difficult to recognize because the symptoms are so variable. If the child refuses to eat solid foods, or has disturbed sleep, or screams at the sight of strangers for example, he may be considered to be neurotic or just going through a temporary emotional crisis. The true meaning of such behavior may go unrecognized for a long time. Types of behavior in an infant or very young child which should be looked upon as danger signals include:

1. If the infant seems strange and "uncuddly" to his mother.
2. Failure to develop loving or affectionate feelings toward their parents or others.
3. Conspicuous placidity, "preferring" to be alone.
4. Stereotyped activities, such as twirling objects.
5. Relates more easily to objects than to people.
6. Does not grasp the meaningful use of objects.
7. An obsessive desire to maintain sameness.
8. Failure to learn to talk.
9. A sudden change in character with symptoms of depression.

There are many theories as to what causes this condition in these children, one theory being that it is the result of a profound disturbance in the parent-child relationship. At present, research has proven one fact: The entire future development of the child is dependent upon a meaningful relationship between the infant and the person caring for him during the first year of life, whether it is the natural mother, foster mother, nurse, technician, or some other person.

The neurotic child, in general, is the one who is always good, overly eager to please everyone in authority, and over-obedient, never rebelling at anything. He is much more considerate of and polite to his elders than is usually considered normal for youngsters. He may worry too much about his lessons and try to be perfect in everything he attempts. His feelings are easier "hurt" and he may even become depressed or unusually sad if he thinks that he has been slighted by the adults who are important to him. Normal youngsters will have a certain amount of arguments and "battles" among themselves, even to the extent of exchanging physical blows. The neurotic child will not fight back; instead, he will run, cry and seek the protection of adults. Because he runs, the other children are only tempted to be even more aggressive toward him. The neurotic child becomes more fearful with an increased tendency to withdraw from any association with other children. The cycle continues until the child succeeds in building up his defenses by maintaining an attitude, which is really a false one, of indifference to the dislike of the others. This in turn appears to be an air of superiority which keeps him isolated and unhappy because the other children dislike him due to this "air." When this piles up in the child's life to the extent that he "can't take it any longer" he may become physically ill, not sleep well and have nightmares, may have a poor appetite with a loss in weight, may be afraid of going outside, and will not want to go to school because he "can't learn anything" due to his inability to concentrate.

Personality disturbances in children which are severe enough to rate a diagnosis of psychosis may occur from about the age of two years and are usually a schizophrenic type of behavior. The most outstanding characteristic of this condition is the child's complete indifference to other children and an apparent lack of feeling for anyone. The child appears withdrawn, isolated and distrustful of everyone. He is so sensitive to rebuff from others that he prefers his own world of dreams rather than to risk being hurt by others by trying to live with them. There may be evidence of sudden phobias. Explosive rages without any apparent reason may occur, such as kicking or striking a younger child, followed by a coldly gleeful type of laugh. The child may then become sullen and speechless, or he may go through a series of queer posturings, muttering and whispering to himself. There may be many disturbances in speech with these children, sometimes being so severe (such as being mute) that they may be thought to be mentally retarded. His speech may be without any meaning at all or without any emotional tone. His personal hygiene and eating habits may be identical with those of a mentally retarded child. All too frequently the child becomes the adult schizophrenic of the hebephrenic type.

Successful treatment of emotionally disturbed children requires care on an individual basis. The therapeutic atmosphere should combine tolerance, firmness, patience and understanding on the part of the nursing personnel caring for them plus an inexhaustible supply of patience. The ward program should be flexible and planned to meet the individual needs of each child.

Another type of disturbed behavior in childhood is the aggressive behavior which if continued into adolescence may be labelled "psychopathic personality disorder" or "incorrigible delinquency."

This behavior is almost the exact opposite of that of the neurotic in that the child is extremely defiant and seemingly unwilling to restrain or control his impulses. He is the bully of the play area and takes advantage of younger children. He may play "hookey" from school, run away from home, become involved in petty robbery or in sexual misbehavior. The child may be alert and even likeable and friendly, but underneath this is a deep distrust that anyone really cares what he feels. There has been nothing in his experience with adults that gives him any reason to love them. Treatment of such a child would, ideally, include the treatment of the parents at the same time.

These few words are but an introduction to the study of the emotional disturbances of childhood.

ROLE OF THE PSYCHIATRIC TECHNICIAN WITH THE WITHDRAWN PATIENT

There are four groupings of symptoms which describe the traditional concept of schizophrenic behavior. It is better to think in terms of *schizophrenic symptoms*, rather than to refer to the patient as a "schizophrenic," because schizophrenia is not a clear-cut disease and the word means different things to different people. Also, the same patient may present different sets of symptoms from one day to the next. However, the clinical "labels" are still necessary in the process of diagnosing (which nursing personnel does not do!)

The person having the *simple* type is not too often committed to a state hospital. They are people who seem to have no ambition and are the "shiftless" type. They are rather dull and rarely seek the company of others. They don't worry about jobs or the future, but are content to let tomorrow take care of itself.

The hebephrenic pattern is the most common of all, making up over one-half of the withdrawn hospitalized patients. The onset is usually in the early teens, one of the first symptoms of peculiar behavior being frequent silly smiling or laughing, for no apparent reason. They tend to withdraw from all normal activities and to regress, or go back to the level of behavior of an infant, to a greater degree than any of the other types.

The *onset of catatonic* behavior may occur quite suddenly, sometimes without any apparent warning signals. The withdrawal occurs in the form of a passive, stuporous state with a tendency to remain in one position for hours at a time. This stuporous condition may, without warning, give way to a state of violent excitement.

The suspicious behavior associated with ideas of being mistreated or of being poisoned, which is typical of the *paranoid* type of withdrawal tends to occur later than the other types, sometimes not showing symptoms until the early thirties.

Although each of the patterns of behavior is specific, they all have *one* feature in common, the attempt by the patient to solve all of life's problems by withdrawing and isolating himself from all social contacts. He will need specialized kinds of attention because he has feelings of terrible loneliness, yet is fearful of any kind of friendship. All nursing care programs must be directed toward preventing the patient from retreating deeper into his world of fantasy and dreams. The development of successful relationships should be based upon acceptance, kind firmness, and consistent friendliness and interest, even though the patient becomes hostile or even makes no response at all.

If the patient can be given treatment during the first six months of his illness and not later than the first year, the prognosis or hope for recovery is usually good. Unfortunately, the well-established routines of a hospital tend to encourage the development of a "chronic" state, especially if the psychiatric technician falls into the trap of looking upon the quiet patient who "causes no trouble" as a "good" patient, and therefore makes no effort to provide variety of any kind to break the deadly monotony.

Communication with the withdrawn patient is difficult to establish. It takes patience and understanding on the part of technician to make contact with a patient who never *appears* to hear or feel. A personal nursing experience of many years ago is as vivid today as it was during the days it occurred, and always reminds me, *never* assume that a patient doesn't hear or know what is going on in his immediate environment: This young woman sat day after day in the same chair in the same location on the ward. She was extremely withdrawn and always sat with her head bowed down upon her chest, her eyes apparently always closed. She never spoke. Somatic therapies such as electro-convulsive treatment or the use of energizers had not yet been introduced. She did not refuse to eat if someone fed her, nor did she soil her clothing if a definite toileting routine was maintained. One of her greatest steps toward recovery was the day she raised her head and called one of the nurses by name! We soon discovered that she could call by their correct name every person who worked on the ward. When asked how she could do this after never having seen any of our faces, she replied "I know your shoes and your voices, and I match them to your face and name! I always looked at your shoes when you walked by me."

If the nursing care is to aid in bringing the withdrawn patient back to reality, then "reality" should be sufficiently interesting to the patient that he will leave his dream world. The process of remotivation takes time but it has proven effective, as evidenced by a report of a patient who after participating in a "remotivation" program after years of hospitalization, left the hospital without permission, and when asked why upon being returned to the hospital said "after hearing all that about S----, I had to go and see for myself."

SUGGESTIONS FOR ESTABLISHING CONTACT WITH REALITY

1. Rebuild patients' self-respect.
   a. Revive an interest in personal appearance. The use of make-up

and care of nails are examples of things that can be done at ward level.
   b. Use of deodorants after bathing.
   c. Encourage patient to wear own clothes.
   d. Retraining in toilet habits may be necessary.
2. Initiate activities and participation in them, by taking part in them with the patients.
   a. Group activities which incorporate outdoor exercise are good.
   b. Use of music, by means of a record player, is often stimulating.
3. Occupational therapy projects in which the patient can use their hands in creating something.
   a. Avoid anything which can become a mechanical repetition.
4. Encourage patients to feed themselves in an adult manner; i.e., see that they get adequate nourishment but do not reinforce their regression by constant spoon-feeding.
5. Make the hospital environment as cheerful and pleasant as possible. This includes what is the most important factor of all; the attitude of the psychiatric technician, which should be one of acceptance, tolerance and understanding of the patient no matter how odd and socially unacceptable his behavior may be.

CARE OF AFFECTIVE, OR MANIC-DEPRESSIVE BEHAVIOR

The psychiatric technician may find it easier to understand the behavior of patients whose actions are described by the terms "manic" or "depressed," because even "normal" people have the experiences of feeling unusually happy (manic) at times as well as having periods of feeling sad, lonely and unwanted (depressed). The technician may also think it more interesting to care for this group of patients for two reasons:

1. They can talk, or communicate, with the patient more readily because what the patient says makes "sense" as opposed to the language of the schizophrenic patient.

2. They can see results from the care which is given the patient in a much shorter time than is true with other mental illnesses.

The manic-depressive psychotic behavior is but an exaggeration of the behavior of the person who has always been very energetic, engages in many community projects, whose disposition may be a combination of lively friendliness and aggressiveness with a tendency to get carried away with himself.

The mental illness consists of a wide swing in mood either toward greatly increased mental and physical activity (*psychomotor hyperactivity*) or greatly decreased mental and physical activity (*psychomotor retardation*). One phase may follow the other, or the individual may have only the increased activity or manic phase, or he may have only the decreased activity or depressed, phase. There is no set time table as to the frequency of occurrence of the episodes, it varies with each patient. (Many years ago I became well acquainted with a patient whose diagnosis was "Manic-depressive psychosis, manic type." When I first met her on the hospital's Receiving Ward, it was her twelfth return to the hospital, in nearly as many years, due to the recurrence of her "manicy" behavior. Her husband stated that he "always knew it was time to get A. back when she started moving all the furniture around in the house, 'cause the next thing would be the breaking up of everything." A. had some insight, or understanding, of her illness and did not resist returning to the hospital. She always seemed to look upon the nursing personnel as friends.)

The manic phase and the depressive phase each have varying degrees of severity in the behavior disturbance of the patient.

THE MANIC PHASE

The range of behavior may be from a *hypomania,* or mild form of increased activity, in which the person may be exceedingly talkative, starts several activities but complete none, considers everyone stupid who does not agree with him and may go on a spending spree, to a more acute form, or even to a state of delirious behavior. In the *acute form,* the psychomotor activities are more intense: the talk is louder, faster and difficult to interrupt, the person may sing loudly, there may be sudden spells of anger, he seems unable to sit still but walks up and down the hallways or around and around in his room, and doesn't have time to sleep, to get a drink of water or to care for his own physical needs. This form of illness may occur suddenly and without any warning signals. The patient who has the delirious type of mania is more mentally confused than in the other types, cannot answer questions and the excited condition is continous, progressing to complete exhaustion unless treated.

ROLE OF THE PSYCHIATRIC TECHNICIAN

The use of the tranquilizing drugs has resulted in a more rapid improvement in the condition of patients suffering from a manic reaction, this in turn making it easier for the psychiatric technician as well as other personnel, to develop positive interpersonnel relationships with the patient. It must be kept in mind however, that the drugs do not cure the patient, but calm him sufficiently to permit other therapies to be of greater benefit to him in less time.

The Attitude of the Psychiatric Technician

These patients, due to their underlying tension and hostility, are not only loud in their speech but are often vulgar and profane, may use sexual words or make seductive gestures toward the nursing personnel of the opposite sex. If the patient chances to observe a "sensitive spot" of the psychiatric technician's such as blemish in the complexion or uneven teeth, he will repeatedly comment about it in an uncomplimentary manner within the hearing of everyone who may be present. The technician must not react in the same manner. The tone of voice which he uses is of utmost importance. A kind voice pitched to a low tone will achieve better results than one with a loud, demanding tone. And never, under any circumstances, shout, curse, or make fun of the patient. Ideally, the psychiatric technician should remain calm in the face of excitement, never show fear when aggressiveness is directed toward him or other patients, does not show embarrassment or concern over the vulgar or obscene expressions of the patient and does not become angry at the patient who directs derogatory remarks toward the technician.

The psychiatric technician should bear in mind that the patient who uses sexually suggestive words or gestures does not necessarily mean that he wishes to indulge in sexual intercourse. He may be seeking reassurance and acceptance, or attempting to reduce his feelings of loneliness, or he may be deliberately trying to upset the employee (especially female) by his behavior, knowing that his behavior will result in a lot of attention being focused upon him. It will be easier to accept such behavior if the technician can look upon it as a plea from the patient for a warm, friendly acceptance, and not that of a personal sexual assault.

It takes time and experience to learn how to adjust and readjust and to develop the appropriate attitudes and approaches to use towards patients. Remember that they are sick and need your care and attention.

Guides to Nursing Care

1. Ward atmosphere should be quiet and non-stimulating.
2. Prevent the hyperactive patient from irritating other patients.
3. Hydrotherapy, such as a continuous tub bath is often beneficial. (This must not be given without a doctor's order.)
4. Programs of recreational and occupational activities should be planned to channel the excessive energy and activity of the patient.
5. Personal attention to meet the physical needs of the patient:
   a. Insure adequate rest.
   b. Insure an adequate intake of fluids and food.
   c. Will need supervision in the care of their skin (bathing), hair, oral hygiene.
   d. Regular toilet schedule is necessary.
   e. Prevention of injuries which may occur as the result of the over-activity.

THE DEPRESSIVE PHASE

In this phase there are also three levels of behavioral symptoms; a simple depression, a more acute expression of the same type of behavior and the most intense type which appears as a stuporous condition.

A mentally and physically depressed (psychomotor retardation) patient is "slowed down" in all of his living processes. He has difficulty in concentrating on anything except his own thoughts of guilt, sinfulness, uselessness and unworthiness in living. He may complain of inability to sleep and of loss of appetite. His physical appearance is one of hopelessness and despair; he sits with head bowed, with a tortured facial expression and his personal hygiene is neglected. His thoughts of himself are self-depreciatory; i.e., he's no good, no one can love him, never has been a success and so on. He assumes the blame for all the problems of the world. It is because of this intense mental torment that he may attempt to kill himself. The suicidal attempt may be with the thought of relieving his unbearable anxiety or it may be for the purpose of atoning for all his sins. (There are many theories as to why people commit suicide which will not be expanded upon here.)

A patient who has an *agitated depression* is emotionally, or mentally, depressed but his physical activities, though limited, are agitated, such as a constant wringing of the hands, all the while pacing back and forth in his room. These patients also tend to be "skin pickers," either of the face or of the hands and arms.

THE ROLE OF THE PSYCHIATRIC TECHNICIAN

Psychiatric treatment of the depressed patient includes the use of drugs and convulsive therapy. Various drugs have been used with considerable differences of opinion as to their success. "Shock" therapy, on the other hand, has proven to be a true miracle-worker in relieving the symptoms of depression. Both metrazol convulsive therapy and electro-convulsive therapy are used; however, electro-shock is most widely used. These treatments "snap" the patient out of his depression, he becomes more optimistic in his outlook on life, and will eat and sleep better. The psychiatric technician may assist the doctor with such treatments, but the important nursing care and program for activities following the treatment involves the technician to a much greater degree.

THE ATTITUDE OF THE PSYCHIATRIC TECHNICIAN

The depressed patient needs reassurance of his worth as a person and that there is someone genuinely interested in him as an individual. A friendly, cheerful approach is desirable, but avoid being too forceful with the cheerfulness; never "force" anything upon a patient. A greeting of "come on and snap out of it, this is a beautiful day!" will many times make the patient seem more unhappy. So too will excessive laughter and joking on the part of the nursing personnel which instead of "cheering" up a depressed patient, will tend to make him more depressed, due in part to his feelings of guilt (because he isn't and cannot feel happy). The psychiatric technician can imply by his own behavior toward the patient that the patient will get well. Take a few minutes, as often as schedules permit, to sit down and talk to the patient. Even though the patient does not converse with you, there is a communication occurring and the patient appreciates the individualized attention. Patience is a necessity when working with the depressed patient because it requires more time to complete the simplest of routines, such as oral hygiene or combing the hair. Use a positive approach in carrying out all nursing care procedures. Part of the treatment of the depressed patient is that of not requiring him to make decisions. Do not ask him, for example, if he "would like to get dressed this morning," but state "Here are your clothes, Mr. (or Mrs.) J---, I'll help you get them on." Never, by word or deed, give the impression that you do not respect the patient for what he is.

Guides to Nursing Care

1. Encourage association with other, active patients.
2. Close attention to physical needs is necessary:
   Toileting schedule to insure proper elimination.
   Personal hygiene: bathing, oral hygiene, hair.
   Personal appearance.
   Adequate intake of food and liquids.
   Keep warm by providing extra clothing, such as a sweater.
   Adequate rest and sleep.
3. Plan a program of activities which will give the patient an opportunity to "work off" his sense of guilt and unworthiness. (The doctor prescribes all such activities.)
4. Plan for activities to stimulate an interest in living.
5. Always remember: *Every depressed patient is a potential suicidal risk.*

PREVENTION OF SUICIDE

The attitude toward the prevention of suicide will vary with the hospital and the needs of the patient. Some hospitals insist on very strict rules and protective measures which results in a prison-like environment. Other hospitals have no established rules, the attitude seeming to be that if a patient is determined to kill himself, there's little that can be done to prevent it. The so-called suicidal precautions in any hospital should be for the purpose of protecting the patient yet be permissive enough to remain therapeutic, not punitive. How this can be carried out is largely dependent upon the psychiatric technician and other nursing personnel.

The establishment of a positive relationship between the patient and a psychiatric technician, or other member of the treatment team, is one of the most effective methods of preventing suicidal attempts. Briefly, a positive relationship means that the technician has made the patient feel that here is someone who cares about him and who is sincerely interested in his welfare; the patient therefore, will not hurt the technician by attempting to kill himself. It will also follow then, that because the technician has this rapport with the patient, he will be able to detect mood changes which provide a cue to the patient's intended behavior, and be able to initiate measures to prevent an attempt at self-destruction. Some of these changes are:

Trouble in sleeping; although the patient goes to sleep without trouble, he will awaken early in the morning and cannot go back to sleep.

A *loss of appetite* will become obvious.

Ability to concentrate, as well as interest in any activity, lessens.

Expression of extreme hopelessness, guilt and self-criticism.

Sudden cheerful mood when there has been no physical treatment to explain the change.

No matter how excellent this relationship may be, many of the so-called standard precautionary measures should not be ignored.

Precautionary Measures

1. Sharp instruments, silverware, manicuring equipment, razors and glassware must be accounted for on all shifts.

Patients must use these under the supervision of nursing personnel.

2. All medicines must be kept behind locked doors, in locked cabinets.

3. When giving medicines, be sure that the patient *swallows* the dose. He may try to accumulate some medicines for suicidal purposes.

4. Many housekeeping supplies, such as insect sprays, lysol, sani-flush or ammonia are poisonous and dangerous. If kept on the ward, keep in a locked cupboard. Do not permit a depressed patient to "help with the cleaning" by giving him a can of Sani-flush and telling him to clean the toilet bowls.

5. Removal of personal possessions such as a belt, neckties, garter belt, bathrobe cords, eyeglasses, watches or articles of clothing from the patient will depend upon the policy of the hospital. Patients have been known to attempt suicide by using any one of these articles, either to hang themselves or to cut blood vessels.

6. Do not assume that because a patient talks about suicide he will not do it. The most casual reference to suicide should be considered a warning and so noted by all nursing personnel.

7. Do not assume that because the depressed patient has improved and seems happy, that the precautions are no longer necessary. This is apt to be the most dangerous period for the patient. It almost seems as though he has made the decision to end his life and is happy and relieved to think that he has made the decision to destroy himself.

8. Any patient who has actually attempted suicide, either before or after admission to the hospital, should be under close observation at all times; when bathing, dressing, toileting, asleep or awake. The degree of "closeness" should be ordered by the doctor, but it would usually mean that the patient is to be within the sight of a member of the nursing staff at all times.

9. Change of shift may provide the moment of relaxed vigilance the patient has been waiting for, just as they may

take advantage of a temporary easing of watchfulness due to less personnel being on duty.

10. When escorting the patient to any activity be alert to the possibility of an attempt on his part to throw himself in front of a passing automobile, or if near water, to pull away from you and attempt to drown himself.

11. Visiting day and visitors result in an increased need for observation of the patient because the visitor may give the patient potentially dangerous articles such as a nail file or a new belt, and if the patient has been taken off the ward for a visit, he may bring in such contraband himself. (A patient in a state hospital once successfully concealed on her person, while out on a visit, a length of rope which was not detected in time to prevent her hanging herself after she was returned to the ward.)

12. It is generally considered more imperative to maintain the "strict" type of precautions where there is inadequate staffing or inexperienced personnel.

THE ELDER CITIZEN OF THE HOSPITAL POPULATION

Individuals over the age of sixty-five years are usually in state mental institutions for one of the following two reasons:

They have grown old during years of hospitalization for a "chronic" mental illness, or, changes in behavior which have been considered unacceptable in their particular social setting, followed up by demands from relatives, or other concerned persons, for restriction of the oldster in a hospital.

These changes in behavior may have been brought on by any one of several factors or combination of circumstances. Often there is not really any sharp change in behavior or mental health; as the person grows older there is just less motivation to keep under control long-standing personality traits that might be considered undesirable. Everyone who lives long enough has to adjust to many changes, but adjustment for too many cannot be achieved in this society of ours, which tries to ignore age.

Some of the major factors that contribute to the development of emotional problems in our senior citizens are social rejection, loss of a spouse, retirement from a job without any interests to take the place of the job, diminution in the circle of friendly associates, feelings of frustration due to failing strength, hearing or sight, a real or imaginary belief that their children have abandoned them and their own sense of self-rejection.

The circumstances related to living conditions, such as having to live in their children's homes, tend to activate *functional* disorders. This may be evidenced by the older person's wandering about the neighborhood because he feels that he no longer has a true part in family life. Regardless of how much children love their parents, it is extremely difficult for two, or three, generations to live in one home. The resulting tensions and difficult personal situations cause the older person to become so emotionally torn that he may develop a functional mental illness with symptoms which appear as severe as if they were the result of organic causes. Their thinking may become so distorted that they may turn against the very persons who care for them the most.

Diseases which cause actual changes in the brain and its functioning, rarely occur before the age of sixty years. The two chief causes are cerebral arteriosclerosis and senile brain disease, or a combination of both. The resulting *organic* mental illness is due to the changes in the blood supply to the brain tissue and in the walls of the blood vessels in the brain. There are two other brain disorders which strike a few years earlier but are rarer, which are related to the aging process: Alzheimer's Disease, which is a presenile condition marked by tiny hardened areas in the brain and by progressive mental weakness and Pick's Disease, which is the result of the atrophy (wasting or diminution in size) of a limited area of the brain.

Besides the various mental states which may occur, such as confusion, agitation, depression, forgetfulness, hallucinations or delusions, organic conditions such as blindness, a paralysis, deafness or a chronic infection may also be present.

The type of behavior of the individual patient will depend upon the sort of person he has been all his life plus the kind of activities he has always pursued. For example, a man who has spent a life time building up a business and has been "the boss" and becomes mentally ill after retiring, will no doubt want to tell everyone how to perform his job and will deeply resent having the psychiatric technician, especially a younger one, telling him what to do. And the woman who has always been "fussy and a worrier" may become agitated and depressed when she no longer has a family to "fuss" over.

The nursing care of any patient with a chronic organic behavior disorder presents a real challenge, but this is especially so with the senile patient. The psychiatric technician who is to work successfully with the elderly patient must first of all have a real feeling of warmth and understanding for the older patients. He must show respect for their years and use their correct name when speaking to the patient. As one elderly gentleman once said when a technician called him "Grandpop," "No young whippersnapper is gonna call me Grandpop, I ain't anybody's Grandpop yet."

The psychiatric technician must be able to accept the idea that it is worthwhile to attempt making life a little happier and more meaningful for these people who in too many instances feel that there is no one in the world who any longer cares about what may happen to them. If the patient is capable of caring for it, he should be permitted to keep in his possession some cherished object, such as a little prayerbook.

A nursing care program for the elderly patient (who may appear to be in his second childhood) closely resembles that which you would plan for retarded children. Such a program should include:

1. Making his environment as hazard free as possible. Remember, their bones are brittle and break easily! *Always* provide adequate assistance when giving tub baths. Eliminate throw rugs and articles of furniture which can be tripped over.
2. Careful attention to personal hygiene. Skin needs special care; avoid drying agents such as alcohol rubs.
3. Keep them warm and out of drafts.
4. A regular routine for activities.
5. Assuring adequate nutrition.
6. May need supervision in toileting.

The psychiatric technician must also bear in mind that rehabilitation therapy such as occupational therapy does not "rehabilitate" in the literal sense. It should be some type of work which not only would "occupy" the patient's time, but should mean something and give a purpose to his life. Music therapy is usually enjoyed by the older patient; in fact, many of them enjoy "peppy" music with a pronounced rhythm. A group of elderly women in one hospital looked eagerly forward to the weekly visit from a younger female patient who came to the ward to play a guitar and sing folk songs to them. The greatest thing the psychiatric technician can do for the "old folks" is to make them feel wanted and useful.

An experiment which is being carried out in a state hospital in California in the admission procedure of patients over the age of sixty-five years is worthy of consideration, in that it encourages the patients to be responsible for their own activities and maintains their self respect.

Both men and women are admitted to the same unit. Separate bathrooms were designated for male and female patients, low beds were installed and there was a noticeable absence of bedside commodes. Every effort was made to duplicate an actual home atmosphere by banishing such sick symbols as wheelchairs. The patients are taught and encouraged to make their own beds, to press their own clothing and to assume as much responsibility as possible for items which have been issued to them. They are encouraged to wear their own clothing, to take daily walks, to visit the canteen and to see movies in the auditorium. Meals are served at small tables, family-style without the use of military-type food trays. Employees serve a meal, if an aged patient desires, and then sit down to eat with the patients. Visitors, especially relatives, are welcome. Visits by patients from other living quarters of the hospital are also permitted.

The initiation of such a program would depend upon the facilities available in an institution, but it tends to eliminate the creation of a feeling of uselessness on the part of the patient, as well as preparing him for future placement in a Family Care program if and when such were available in the community.

Meanwhile, no one can go wrong by giving an old person the benefit of the doubt that his condition might be improved by providing him with interests and a reason for living but putting no more pressure on him than he can comfortably take.

ALCOHOLISM, OR CARE OF THE PROBLEM DRINKER

The drinking person can easily discover for himself at what stage he is on the way to becoming an alcoholic. Honest self-evaluation should enable anyone to see if he is headed for trouble.

The person who becomes addicted to the use of alcohol is usually one who has many deep-seated emotional conflicts, who suffer from feelings of inferiority, and who is anxious and lonely. Curious experimenting soon leads to choice of favorite drinks that may be enjoyed with friends at business or social functions. There is a steady progression from this social drinking, to that which eases the pressures of the job, or to relieve boredom, to that which compensates for inability to achieve personal success and fulfillment. Whatever their rationalization may be, the alcohol inhibits certain centers in the brain and the individual will be able to express himself in words and actions which otherwise he would not be able to.

The problem drinker seems to be determined to ruin not only his own life but his family with him; his drink is more important than is food for his children. He makes all kinds of excuses for his drinking, all of which are a cover-up for his feelings of inadequacy. The earlier in life the use of alcohol becomes a problem, the more difficult it is to treat.

The belief that so potent a liquid as alcohol must be capable of causing serious disease is an old one. Dr. Benjamin Rush stated many years ago that "ardent spirits" dispose the body "to every form of acute disease; they moreover excite fevers in persons predisposed to them, from other causes."* Twentieth century research tends to soften alcohol's image somewhat, even though it does not create the image of alcohol as being benign and milk like. Alcohol is implicated in a number of varied diseases but in most cases it plays an indirect role. Disease and/or conditions such as general malnutrition, vitamin deficiency diseases, liver cirrhosis and nervous and mental conditions are frequently found in alcoholics, but are not peculiar to them alone.

The most frequent cause for admission of an alcoholic to a hospital is the "shakes"—a state of tremulousness often combined with general irritability, nausea and vomiting. Delirium tremens appears

---

*Roche Laboratories, Division of Hoffman-LaRoche, Inc.: *Aspects on Alcoholism,* Nutley, N. J., Roche Laboratories, 1964.

to be a much severer form of this condition. Usually by the time the individual is admitted to the hospital he will need a concentrated program of rehabilitation, vitamin and diet therapy, special attention to personal hygiene and encouragement of an interest in his personal appearance. If he is confused and disoriented he will need to be protected from possible self-injury. The distressing withdrawal symptoms demand expert medical attention and management of these conditions follows well-known patterns. They are a far cry from treatments prescribed by Dr. Rush; among other "remedies" he suggested "thrusting a feather down the patient's throat to induce vomiting, plunging him into cold water, or terrifying him into sobriety."* Modern treatment methods utilize a vast array of psychopharmaceuticals for the relief of anxiety, tension, tremor and the inability to sleep, all of which are suffered in some degree by the alcoholic undergoing treatment.

After the alcoholic patient has recovered from the acute period of his illness, the attitudes of the treatment personnel, including that of the psychiatric technician is all important. Trained staff can relate to patients with understanding, confidence and respect. These attitudes are double-edged and almost without exception, the patient will respond in kind with the behavior expected of them. Many of these patients are outwardly very charming, pleasant individuals and the inexperienced employee will be manipulated, or "used" by the patient to meet his needs, instead of the employee being the leader. The patient tends to have a superior attitude toward the "mentals" who may be in the same area, not considering himself as sick as the latter are. The technician should tactfully encourage the patient to take part in group activities.

Generally speaking, neither medical nor psychiatric methods of treatment have "cured" the alcoholic; drugs such as Antabuse, the conditioned reflex method and electro-shock treatments have all been used. The most successful "treatment" is a form of group psychotherapy as practiced by Alcoholics Anonymous. The members of any one group are individuals who, in most cases, have had some form of treatment for their problem drinking and join the organization voluntarily. The twelve steps of A.A. are based upon the

*Roche Laboratories, Division of Hoffman-LaRoche, Inc.: *Aspects on Alcoholism,* Nutley, N. J., Roche Laboratories, 1964.

concept that the individual is unable to help himself and needs to ask for help from God, followed by group support to control his drinking. The first step which must be hurdled is admission upon the person's part that he is an alcohol addict. When, or if, the person feels himself slipping in his decision not to drink, he may call upon a member of his group at any time of the day or night for help. The individual has reached the twelfth step when he expresses a desire to aid another alcoholic when called upon for assistance.

CARE OF PATIENTS WHO HAVE BECOME ADDICTED TO DRUGS

Narcotics addiction is a growing problem of modern civilization and there are many inconsistencies in available statistics. F.B.I. Director J. Edgar Hoover has been quoted as saying "Our files contain not one single case of proven cure for heroin addiction. There is no release but death." Narcotic addiction is a psychiatric, medical, social and legal problem.

Reasons for individuals to start on the road to addiction are as varied and many as are the individuals. The drug provides a "booster" to the emotionally unstable person which gets him through the tension-filled society of today; or it provides a certain status in an adolescent's group, or the beginning is due to curiosity as to just what the effect will be; or drugs may be taken out of rebellion against society. There is also the legal addict, i.e., the person who during the course of hospitalization for surgical or other treatment has become addicted to a drug which was used for the relief of pain and because the patient has an already existing condition such as a congenitally weak heart, the physician decides that it would be dangerous to the welfare of the patient to discontinue the use of the addicting drug. After discharge from the hospital, such an individual receives his prescribed drug from his physician at designated intervals. Such a "legal" addict carries identification (of the medical situation) at all times.

Most narcotic addicts who are committed to a state hospital have already gone through withdrawal symptoms. If patients are admitted who are undergoing withdrawal symptoms, various types of physiological supportive treatment is given. The drug "methadone" may be used in diminishing amounts to control the withdrawal symptoms.

There is no specific treatment for narcotic addiction, but after the withdrawal phase of physical treatment has been accomplished, other forms of therapy is initiated.

The psychiatric approach is based on the assumption that the addiction is symptomatic of a mental or personality disorder, and therefore treatment can be successful if the mental processes or personality disorder can be modified through therapy. The first treatment required in many cases is of a physical nature, to correct the serious physical and nutritional deficiencies often seen in these individuals. Continuing therapy then takes many forms and should be individualized as much as possible. The kinds of therapy used include group psychotherapy, individual therapy, vocational rehabilitation, and individual counseling with various members of the hospital's professional staff, depending upon the needs of the individual patient. Such professional counselors might include other than a psychiatrist, psychologists, psychiatric social workers, chaplains, vocational rehabilitation counselors or nursing personnel. Meeting regularly with other individuals having problems of narcotic addiction is often helpful in assisting the patient to a better understanding of his own problems. In the hospital he is given an opportunity for introspection, sound professional guidance, and the development of regular habits of living and socialization.

The second and most important phase of the treatment is the post-hospital treatment. Here the patient has opportunity to continue the treatment processes in a manner that can really test his progress. While receiving treatment as an out-patient he can again become a productive member of society and this, in itself, is helpful. Regular interviews with his therapist are essential and occasionally it may be necessary for him to return to the hospital when the demands of his environment become too stressful. The therapist must be in a position to work with the patient's environment as well as with the patient himself, and it may even be further necessary to change the patient's residence. It is usually necessary to work with the patient's family and sometimes with his employers and friends so that they may be in a position to assist in the rehabilitation processes as well as to understand their role in the patient's illness.

Perhaps even more of a social and legal problem is that of the use of the non-narcotic habit-forming drugs, such as the barbiturates. In general, however, the underlying reasons for the person to resort to their use are basically the same just as the basic treatment philosophies are the same.

The State of California has been in the process of pioneering a Narcotic Addict Control Plan which provides treatment for men and women and is designed to get the addict off the street, thus reducing addiction through association. There is no broad basis of treatment and no specific line of correction which may be said to be generally successful. The Rehabilitation Center provides treatment and control based on today's knowledge of the addict:

1. Compulsory, continued treatment in a drug free environment for a minimum period, at least six months.

2. Follow-up out-patient supervision and help after return to the home environment.

3. Anti-narcotic testing, then further treatment in the Center if the addict is detected using drugs again.

CARE OF THE SOCIOPATHIC PERSONALITY BEHAVIOR DISORDERS

Only a small percentage of the people who have such disorders ever get to a psychiatric hospital for treatment. There is a general lack of agreement among therapists as to how to treat such disturbances.

The sociopath's symptoms show up as disturbances in their social relations or in their behavior toward society. They cannot be depended upon on a job, they are frequently dishonest, often are unfaithful to their spouse, and steals whenever he feels like it even when he knows that he will be detected. He has no real liking or affection for anyone and lives only for the present. Also included among the undesirable traits the sociopath may have are a variety of perversions which are evidenced by antisocial moral and sexual behavior. Most of the episodes of "abnormal" sexual behavior are the manifestation, upon the part of the individual, of immaturity in obtaining sexual gratification. There are various types of sexual perversions, but homosexuality (sexual attachment and love for a person of the same sex) is the one which receives the most attention in our society.

What causes the development of such imperfect relationships is not clearly understood. The psychoanalysts have developed many theories, one being that the adult's behavior is the result of severe disturbances occurring in the earliest psychosexual development of the child. Some authorities even deny the existence of the sociopath as such.

It matters not how much or what type of punishment is handed out to him, he does not gain any benefit from it; neither does he modify his behavior as a result of his mistakes.

When you first come in contact with an individual who has been hospitalized because of such antisocial behavior, you no doubt will question *why* this person is in the hospital; he seems so normal. In general, the patient is a smooth talker, gives the impression of having above average intelligence, (and he may have), may be attractive in his personal appearance, and will play upon the sympathies of those who are caring for him. The psychiatric technician, as well as the professional nurse, must bear in mind that no patient is *kept* in a psychiatric hospital unless he is mentally ill.

Historically, society's attitude toward the behavior of the sociopath, the sexual psychopath in particular, has been punitive with imprisonment being the only way to handle the problem. A fresh approach in handling sexual psychopathy, that of therapy, is being carried out at the Atascadero State Hospital in California. As a part of the therapeutic program, social therapy in the form of patient government is accepted as part of the hospital's administrative pattern. The fact that most of the patients are court committed for indefinite periods of time would not ordinarily be conducive to an optimistic treatment program. The patient inspired program has initiated many occupational and recreational projects. All of the patients have shown an interest in learning all they can about the various aspects of their illness, and on different occasions have invited well-known authorities on law and criminology and social scientists to meet with them for discussion on the subject of sexual deviations. The patients in turn give educational talks to visiting professional groups.

The psychiatric technician should avoid being "taken in" by the manipulations of the patient, yet at the same time letting the patient know that he is being accepted as he is. The sociopath likes to identify himself with the nursing personnel but this should, in most cases, be discouraged with a quiet but firm insistance that the patient conform with the regulations. Limits must be set upon his behavior, and whenever the patient exhibits antisocial behavior, you must treat him in such a way that he will know that you want to help him even though he cannot be permitted to continue such behavior. A temper tantrum is an example of the type of behavior which such a patient may display, or he may indulge in an episode of destroying some of the ward's furnishings. The psychiatric technician who is faced with such a nursing care problem should call for assistance before attempting to control the patient.

The patient with antisocial behavior frequently asks for special privileges, (especially of an employee who may be newly assigned to the ward) such as permission to go off the ward for what would ordinarily be considered a quite legitimate reason—but—*caution*; check your patient's orders sheet or chart! In general, these patients are unreliable and if there are no written orders granting special privileges, you may have an unauthorized vacancy to account for.

These patients vary greatly in regards to their emotional needs but like everyone else, they thrive on praise and recognition for acceptable performance and behavior. Remember, scolding or lecturing serves no useful purpose with the sociopath; it only makes him angry.

MODIFICATION OF BASIC NURSING PROCEDURES

All procedures are carried out in a manner which can best meet the needs of the patient. By the act of being admitted to a psychiatric hospital, it is implied that the individual is not capable of assuming responsibility for his actions. He may not want to cooperate with any request; he may express thoughts of killing himself; he may refuse to eat; he may be so hyperactive that he has no "time" for treatments; or he may be frightened of the strange environment.

In general, the modification of nursing procedures will depend upon the principles which underlie the procedure which is to be carried out and upon the degree of cooperation which can be expected from the patient. Too many times under the pressure of work load and the desire to get everything done before it is time to go off duty, the psychiatric technician or nurse tends to lose sight of the responsibility of caring for the patient as a PERSON. Therefore, modifications of nursing procedures should be done with the first consideration being given to the emotional response of the patient, at the same time striving for the desired results.

Every patient *deserves an explanation* of any treatment which is to be given him. Such a matter as a ward's activities schedule requires an explanation as to its necessity to the newly admitted patient. This is especially true if it be a person who considers conformation to any set of rules and regulations to be ridiculous!

If a patient's cooperation cannot be gained, do not attempt to carry out any procedure without securing adequate assistance. Many times the mere presence of a second nursing person encourages the patient to be more cooperative. The actual use of force in attempting to carry out a procedure only tends to nullify the therapeutic results desired.

A minimum amount of equipment, to satisfactorily perform the procedures, is desirable as there is then less opportunity for damage if the patient should react impulsively or aggressively.

Temperatures are usually taken by rectum with the thermometer being held by the psychiatric technician or nurse. It is not only considered the most accurate method but this technique protects the patient from possible self-injury. However, this procedure as well as vaginal douching for female patients and the administration of an enema may be looked upon as a sexual assault upon their person by certain types of patients. Be alert to this type of emotional response and do not attempt to force the procedure upon the patient. The doctor may order a modification of the necessary procedure or he may instruct that nothing be done for a specified period of time.

An adequate intake of food is important for every patient. However, there are many reasons why a patient may refuse food: voices (hallucinations) are telling him not to eat, he may be afraid of being poisoned, or he may be so depressed that he cannot feed himself.

The psychiatric technician or nurse may have to be very permissive and spoon feed the patient, instead of using useless verbal repetition and admonitions to eat. A suspicious patient may be convinced that the food is not poisoned if the nursing person will first taste or drink some of the offered food. If all nursing procedures fail, it will depend upon the doctor as to how long the patient is to be permitted to go without nourishment. The patient may then be fed by nasal gavage or intravenous feeding.

The amount of responsibility given the psychiatric technician pertaining to the administration of medications will depend upon the hospital and the doctor. Medications should never in any instance be left sitting around the ward, unattended, to be given at a later time. Paper cups are not only very convenient to use in dispensing medicines to patients but also eliminate all the possible safety hazards associated with the use of glass or metal cups. Plastic cups are also safe to use. After the patient has taken the medicine, the nursing person must be sure that the patient has swallowed the dose, even if this requires the inspection of the inside of the patient's mouth. A patient who has suicidal tendencies may attempt to collect enough medication of a specific kind for a lethal dose by attempting to "hide" a pill or capsule under the tongue or in the inside of the cheek, swallow the water which is given him with which to take the medicine, and when you leave his side, remove the medicine to hoard for future use. Once again, treat the patient with respect and as a person, but be alert to his emotional responses.

Bathing and showering is usually done under the supervision of an employee. The degree of observation and supervision is dependent upon the type of patient. A patient who has a history of suicidal attempts, for example, should not be left in a bathroom unattended. An elderly, feeble patient needs much the same personal assistance that you would give a child.

Sterile procedures, such as catheterization or the changing of a surgical dressing, cannot be modified to anything other than sterile. If the patient will not cooperate, adequate assistance must be obtained to restrain the patient manually until completion of the procedure. When it is time to retire for the night a patient may not want to go to bed in a dark room. His fear of the dark, while you may not understand the reason for it, is very real to the patient, and he wants the light left on. Even though the ward may have a "rule" which states that *all* lights must be out by a specific hour, a modification of the "rule" will result in a patient going to sleep without needing a sedative or perhaps requiring restraint.

SELECTED READING

Many books, pamphlets and articles have been published on the subjects of mental retardation and mental illness. This brief listing has been compiled for the benefit of the student or for the individual who is not acquainted with the availability of material, to aid them in selecting subjects with which to broaden and enrich their knowledge and understanding.

BOOKS

Anthony, Catherine Parker: *Textbook of Anatomy and Physiology, 6th ed.* St. Louis, Mosby, 1963.

Armstrong, I. L., and Browder, J. J.: *The Nursing Care of Children.* Philadelphia, Davis, 1958.

Battista, O. A.: *Mental Drugs: Chemistry's Challenge to Psychosurgery.* Philadelphia and New York, Chilton, 1960.

Beers, Clifford: *A Mind That Found Itself.* Garden City, Doubleday, 1953.

Blodgett, Harriett E., and Warfield, Grace J.: *Understanding Mentally Retarded Children.* New York, Appleton, 1959.

Brown, Martha M., and Fowler, Grace R.: *Psychodynamic Nursing.* Philadelphia and London, Saunders, 1954.

Buck, Pearl S.: *The Child Who Never Grew.* New York, Day, 1950.

Caplan, Gerald: *Emotional Problems of Childhood.* New York, Basic Books, 1955.

Cardwell, Viola E.: *Cerebral Palsy: Advances in Understanding and Care.* New York, North River Press, 1956.

Copa, Cornell, and Pines, Maya: *Retarded Children Can Be Helped.* Great Neck, Channel Press, 1957.

DeMartino, Manfred F., and Stacey, Chalmers L.: *Counseling and Psychotherapy with the Mentally Retarded.* Glencoe, Free Press, 1957.

Deutsch, A.: *The Mentally Ill in America, 2nd ed.* New York, Columbia Univ. Press, 1952.

Fitzsimmons, Laura: *Textbook for Psychiatric Attendants.* New York, Macmillan, 1953.

French, Edw. L., and Scott, J. Clifford: *Child in the Shadows, A Manual for Parents of Retarded Children.* New York, Lippincott, 1960.

Ginott, Haim G.: *Group Psychotherapy with Children.* New York McGraw-Hill, 1961.

Heiser, Karl F.: *Our Backward Children*. New York, Norton, 1955.

Ilg, Frances, and Ames, Louise Bates: *The Gesell Institutes Child Behavior*. New York, Dell, 1960.

Ingram, Madelene E.: *Principles of Psychiatric Nursing, 4th ed*. Philadelphia, Saunders, 1948.

Junker, Karen Stensland: *The Child in the Glass Ball*. New York, Abingdon Press, 1964.

Kalkman, Marion E.: *Introduction to Psychiatric Nursing, 2nd ed*. New York, McGraw-Hill, Blakiston, 1958.

Kanner, Leo: *Child Psychiatry, 2nd ed*. Springfield, Thomas, 1955.

Kanner, Leo: *A History of the Care and Study of the Mentally Retarded*. Springfield, Thomas, 1964.

Kirk, Samuel, Karnes, M. B., and Kirk, Winifred: *You and Your Retarded Child*. New York, MacMillan, 1955.

Krug, Elsie: *Pharmacology in Nursing*. St. Louis, Mosby, 1963.

Levinson, Abraham: *The Mentally Retarded Child*. New York, Day, 1952.

Martin, Wm. E., and Stindler, Celia Burns: *Child Behavior and Development*. New York, Harcourt, 1959.

Mary Theodore, Sister: *The Challenge of the Retarded Child*. Milwaukee, Bruce, 1959.

Matheny, Ruth V., and Topalis, Mary: *Psychiatric Nursing, 3rd ed*. St. Louis, Mosby, 1961.

Menninger, Karl A.: *Man Against Himself*. New York, Harcourt, 1939.

Menninger, Karl A.: *The Vital Balance*. New York, Viking, 1963.

Menninger, Karl A., and Leaf, Munro: *You and Psychiatry*. New York, Scribner, 1955.

Mereness, Dorothy, and Karnosh, Louis J.: *Essentials of Psychiatric Nursing, 6th ed*. St. Louis, Mosby, 1962.

Mezer, Robert R., M.D.: *Dynamic Psychiatry in Simple Terms*. New York, Springer, 1956.

Murry, Dorothy G.: *This Is Stevie's Story*. Elgin, Brethern, 1956.

Peplau, Hildegard: *Interpersonal Relations in Nursing*. New York, Putnam, 1952.

Peterson, Sigurd: *Retarded Children: God's Children*. Philadelphia, Westminster, 1960.

Rapier, Koch, Moran, Geronsin, Cady, and Jensen: *Practical Nursing, 2nd ed*. St. Louis, Mosby, 1962.

Rosenzweig, L. E., and Long, Julia: *Understanding and Teaching the Dependent Retarded Child*. Darien, Educational, 1960.

Ruesch, Jurgen, M.D., and Bateson, Gregory: *Communication, the So-*

cial Matrix of Psychiatry. New York, Norton, 1951.

Sarason, S. B.: *Psychological Problems in Mental Deficiency, 3rd ed.* New York, Harper, 1959.

Sellew, Gladys, and Pepper, Mary: *Nursing of Children, 7th ed.* Philadelphia, Saunders, 1953.

Steele, Katharine M., and Manfreda, M. L.: *Psychiatric Nursing, 6th ed.* Philadelphia, Davis, 1959.

Watson, E. H., and Lowrey, George H.: *Growth and Development of Children, 3rd ed.* Chicago, Yr. Bk. Pub., 1958.

Weiss, Madeline O.: *Attitudes in Psychiatric Nursing.* New York, Putnam, 1954.

PAMPHLETS

Dittman, Laura: *The Mentally Retarded Child at Home: A Manual for Parents.* Children's Bureau, U. S. Department of Health, Education and Welfare, Washington, D. C., 1959.

Dybwad, Gunner: *Not all of One Mold.* International Journal of Religious Education, vol. 36, No. 9, May, 1961.

Haynes, Una, R.N.: *The Role of Nursing in Programs for Patients with Cerebral Palsy and Related Disorders.* United Cerebral Palsy Associations, Inc., New York, May, 1962.

Saltman, Jules: *Meeting the Challenge of Cerebral Palsy.* Public Affairs Pamphlet No. 158B, United Cerebral Palsy Associations, Inc., New York, January, 1964.

The National Council for Retarded Children, Inc., 386 Park Avenue South, New York 16, N. Y., has listings of many pamphlets of interest to those working in the field of mental retardation. A few suggestions, all of which may be obtained from the above address, are:

A New Dimension of Love: The story of a young couple who became the parents of a mongoloid child and how they faced the situation.

Holy Communion for the Mentally Retarded Child: Francis J. Connell, C.SS.R., answers to questions on the subject of eligibility of the child to receive the sacrament.

How Retarded Children Can Be Helped: Evelyn Hart, a public affairs pamphlet.

Needs of Parents of Mentally Retarded Children: Mrs. Max A. Murry, six major problems faced by parents of retarded children are related to the need for counseling.

Punching Holes in the Dark: Dorothy G. Murray, Vice President, South East Region, National Association for Retarded Children, 1965.

Stevie's Teacher: Evelyn F. MacGowan, an inspiring story of one teach-

214 *Practical Care of the Mentally Retarded and Mentally Ill*

er's efforts with a retarded pupil in a regular kindergarten.

The Child Who Is Mentally Retarded: W. S. Children's Bureau.

The Mentally Retarded and the Church: Marion O. Lerrigo, Ph.D.; a Protestant overview.

The Three R's for the Retarded: Naomi H. Chamberlin, and Dorothy Moss.

Will My Baby be Born Normal? Joan Gould, a public affairs pamphlet dealing with genetics and eugenics.

Windows of Understanding: NARC's reading list especially selected for parents who are newly faced with the discovery of mental retardation in their child.

ARTICLES

Bartman, Richard E.: *Our neglected problem: Psychiatric Treatment for the mentally retarded. Mental Hospitals,* 1:46-47, September, 1960.

Dittman, Laura: *Home training for retarded children. Children,* May-June, 1957, pp. 89-94.

McCormick, Elsie: *New hope for darkened minds. Reader's Digest Association.* Pleasantville, New York, March, 1962.

Penny, Ruthanna, and Mittelberg, Wilma: *36 Cafeterias. Mental Hospitals,* 11:8-36, American Psychiatric Association, Washington, D. C., October, 1960.

Penny, Ruthanna: *Idiots are human beings or meeting the social needs of the profoundly mentally retarded patient.* Paper presented at 120th Annual Meeting of the American Psychiatric Association and published in summary form, A.P.A., Washington, D. C., May, 1964.

Penny, Ruthanna: *Everything from A to Z. Staff,* 1:3-8, American Psychiatric Association, Washington, D. C., Fall, 1964.

Penny, Ruthanna: *Needed: Substitute parents or training the profoundly mentally retarded patient for return to the community.* Paper prepared for the 121st Annual Meeting of the American Psychiatric Association and published in summary form, A.P.A., Washington, D. C., May, 1965.

Robinson, Alice M.: *Remotivation Technique,* Smith Kline and French Laboratories, Mental Health Education Unit, Philadelphia, 1959.

Rosenzweig, Louis: *How far have we come? American Journal of Mental Deficiency.* 64:1-18, July, 1959.

Shelton, J. T., M.D., Mittelberg, Wilma, and Penny, Ruthanna: *Come and get it! Food Talks.* Nutrition Services Section, Department of Mental Hygiene, Sacramento, California, April, 1963.

Wright, Margaret, et al: *Series on Mental Retardation, American Journal of Nursing,* September, 1963, pp. 70-82.

BIBLIOGRAPHY

Armstrong, I. L., and Browder, J. J.: *The Nursing Care of Children*. Philadelphia, Davis, 1958.

Blodgett, Harriett E., and Warfield, Grace J.: *Understanding Mentally Retarded Children*. New York, Appleton, 1959.

Brown, Martha M., and Fowler, Grace R.: *Psychodynamic Nursing*. Philadelphia, Saunders, 1954.

Cardwell, Viola E.: *Cerebral Palsy; Advances in Understanding and Care*. New York, The North River Press, Inc., 1956.

DeMartino, M. F., and Stacey, C. L.: *Counseling and Psychotherapy with the Mentally Retarded*. Glencoe, The Free Press, 1957.

Department of National Health and Welfare, Mental Health Division: *The Backward Child*. Ottawa, 1952.

Department of Mental Hygiene: *State School Training Manual—Attendants*. New York, 1959.

Deutsch, A.: *The Mentally Ill in America, 2nd ed.* New York, Columbia Univ. Press, 1952.

DiMichael, S. G., Editor: *Vocational Rehabilitation of the Mentally Retarded*. Washington, D. C., U. S. Dept. of Health, Education and Welfare, Rehabilitation Service Series, Booklet No. 123, p. 101-102.

Fitzsimmons, Laura: *Textbook for Psychiatric Attendants*. New York, MacMillan Co., 1953.

Ginott, H. G.: *Group Psychotherapy with Children*. New York, McGraw-Hill, 1961.

Heiser, Karl F.: *Our Backward Children*. New York, Norton, 1953.

Ingram, Madelene E.: *Principles and Techniques of Psychiatric Nursing, 4th ed.* Philadelphia, Saunders, 1948.

Levinson, Abraham, M.D.: *The Mentally Retarded Child: A Guide for Parents*. New York, Day, 1952.

Matheny, Ruth V., and Topalis, Mary: *Psychiatric Nursing, 3rd ed.* St. Louis, Mosby, 1961.

Mereness, Dorothy, and Karnosh, L. J.: *Psychiatry for Nurses, 6th ed.* St. Louis, Mosby, 1962.

National Lutheran Council, Division of Welfare: *The Church and the Mentally Retarded*. New York, 1961.

215

Porterville State Hospital: *Administrative Manual.* Porterville, 1965.

Rapier, Koch, Moran, Fleming, Cady, and Jenson: *Practical Nursing.* St. Louis, Mosby, 1958, Chap. 35-38.

Rodman, Charlotte R.: *A Guide for Psychiatric Aides.* New York, Mac-Millan, 1956.

Rosenzweig, L. E., and Long, Julia: *Understanding and Teaching the Dependent Retarded Child.* Darien, Educational Publishing Corp., 1960.

Sarason, S. B.: *Psychological Problems in Mental Deficiency, 3rd ed.* New York, Harper, 1959.

Sellew, Gladys, and Pepper, Mary: *Nursing of Children, 7th ed.* Philadelphia, Saunders, 1953.

Steele, K. M., and Manfreda, M.: *Psychiatric Nursing, 6th ed.* Philadelphia, Davis, 1959.

Watson, E. H., and Lowry, George H.: *Growth and Development of Children, 3rd ed.* Chicago, Yr. Bk. Pub., 1958.

Weiss, Madeline: *Attitudes in Psychiatric Nursing Care, 3rd ed.* New York, Putnam, 1954.

APPENDICES

Appendix A

WARD ACTIVITIES HANDBOOK*

A handbook such as this one, is the work of many people and many departments. Ideas, projects, games and activities must be compiled from various sources. Nursing Services, as well as the School, has contributed much.

Many books, periodicals, journals and other media have been combed to bring out in this handbook those suggested activities we feel are the most likely to succeed with mentally retarded patients.

Anyone who has contact with the patient shares, to some extent, a responsibility for patient activities. However, Nursing Services with its twenty-four hour patient contact carries the largest responsibility for those activities occurring on or about the ward.

This handbook, therefore, is published primarily for ward personnel: the Psychiatric Technician Trainee, the Technician, the Technician I and Technician II. Many hospital personnel in classifications other than these can, however, benefit from various portions of this handbook.

INITIATING AN ACTIVITIES PROGRAM ON THE WARDS

Try these activities . . . some will work with your group, some will not; some will work with a group one day and not the next. All you can do is *try* them and see.

Activities will not do the impossible . . . there is no magic word or game that will suddenly quiet your patients or make your quiet patients jump up and play. The most important single thing that

*Porterville State Hospital, Porterville, California. James T. Shelton, M.D., Superintendent and Medical Director. Prepared by Rehabilitation Therapies Department, Milt M. Hustad Supervisor of Rehabilitation Therapies.

will determine the success or failure of an activities program in your building is your *attitude.* If you can show genuine interest in the children and in the game or activity you are trying to put across, the battle is won! A part of this overall picture is the importance of a friendly, understanding and firm attitude toward the child. Be alert to each child . . . find out who the shy ones are and who are the leaders. Try to learn what each child likes and can do in the line of activities.

It is physically impossible for a therapist, teacher or supervisor to be at all the wards at all times. Therefore, if activities are to take place on the ward, *you* must help to initiate them. Use the therapists as consultants; ask them for new games to play, ideas for new activities, help in how to handle a certain group; give them suggestions for play equipment you think your children could use; tell him when activities conflict with ward work and what you suggest as a change . . . use them in any way that will make your job of handling activities easier!

Some approaches you can use to the child in presenting activities are:

Repetition. Don't expect the child to understand the first time through; repeat and repeat.

Imitation. Don't tell him how to do or play something, show him!

Praise. Be sure to praise the child for something he has done well according to his ability.

Remember that each of these children is different in their likes and dislikes of certain activities as well as in other areas. Ideally we should try to have a program to fit the child *not* fit the child into the program.

There Are Certain Methods of Control That You Might Try If Certain Patients Are Disrupting the Activity

1. Speaking repeatedly to the child.
2. Redirecting his interest to something else.
3. Isolating the child from the rest of the group.
4. Depriving the child of the activity.

You Will Have Success with the Activities You Lead If You Split Your Group

Try a smaller group of patients first—the others will join in the activity as they become interested.

Know How to Play the Game

Understand the activity or game yourself before you try to teach it.

Get the Attention of the Group

Before you start explaining; speak where everyone can see you; speak to be heard but do not shout.

Demonstrate the Activity

Before playing it, make sure that all understand how to play.

Play in the Game Yourself

If possible; interest in the activity will lag if you just give directions and then stand aside.

Keep Things Moving

All the time; use variations of game being played; follow thru on same formations if possible (line games together, circle, etc.)

Stop a Game at Peak

Of interest, not after children tire of it.

Vary the Games Played

Alternate the activities as to active, quiet, etc.

Learn to Adapt Activities

To your children's level, make a game simpler or more difficult according to the children; make an active circle game into a quiet one by just having children sit in a circle; think up new games or variations as you go along.

Try to Teach Games Children Can Play by Themselves

When you are not there; our patients can learn many games that they will play among themselves.

Use Recognized Leaders Within the Patient Group

Every ward has one, two or three ringleaders that the group as a whole will follow; get to know these leaders and use them to help.

Recognize That These Children Are Different

In their play and adapt accordingly; if everyone wants to be "IT", go along with them and choose someone to be "not it", etc.

PRIMARY ACTIVITIES

Walking

Walking within a given area on ward

Walks on grounds

Follow the Leader (walking)—Following a person (patient or employee) in various simple maneuvers around the ward or area.

Marching Single File—without music.

Variation: with music.

Variation: around chairs or designated objects.

Marching with Partners: Two by two.

Play Train—Line up chairs.

Variation: children line up chairs.

Variation: children make train sounds and motions.

Variation: children walk, pushing chairs in single line make train sounds.

On and Off Game—Blanket or chalked area of similar size—Children instructed "On Blanket." When everyone is on then "Off Blanket."

Follow the Leader (Directions)—Technician faces groups and performs simple movements which are followed by patients.

Example: Clapping hands, raising arms over head, raising arms to shoulders, jumping in place, turning around, etc.

Follow the Leader (By signs)—Come here—Stop—Sit down—Stand up—Go back, etc.

Paper Tears—Technician directs children in simple tearing of paper into halves, quarters, strips, etc.

Paper Crumple—Crumpling newspaper into balls and throwing into some predetermined place, preferably in wastebasket.

Paper Pick-up—Logically follows the two previous activities. Waste containers set in middle of area and children follow technician's example of picking up paper and depositing in a container.

Musical activities—Clapping to music—rocking doll to music, swaying in rhythmic fashion, outstretched arms to fly as birds.

SECONDARY ACTIVITIES

"Good Morning"

"Good Afternoon"

Technician clasps patient's hand and says "Good morning" to him. Patient clasps technician's right hand and says "Good morning" to him. Patient clasps patient's right hand and says "Good morning" to him.

Ring Around the Rosey

Ring around the rosey

Pockets full of posey

Ashes, ashes

All fall down

Children form in circle holding hands, singing, and marching or skipping to the left or right. Upon singing "All fall down", sit down or squat.

Gallant Ship

Three times around went the gallant ship

Three times around went she

Three times around went the gallant ship

Then she sank to the bottom of the sea

Children in circle, facing in, hold hands singing, marching or skipping to the left or right. When "Sank to the bottom of the sea" is sung, children squat.

Sally Go Round the Moon

Sally go round the stars

Sally go round the moon

Sally go round the chimney pots

Sunday afternoon—"Whoops"!

Children in circle, facing in, holding hands, singing, and marching or skipping to the left or right, when "Whoop" is chanted, children squat clap hands over head.

Story Telling

Children seated in semi-circle around technician who presents large picture of familiar objects to group. Technician identifies objects one at a time to each child individually. Then technician brings objects together in telling a *short* story. Children participate by recognition of objects in following manner:

Variation: Children point to objects at direction of technician.

Variation: Children point to objects and call out names at direction of technician.

Rolling the Ball

Children sit or stand in lines or in circle and roll ball (large, rubber).

Variation: Patient rolls ball in any direction.

Variation: Patient rolls ball in given direction.

Variation: Patient rolls ball at a given target.

Bead Stringing

Patient strings beads.

Variation: Patient strings series of beads copying pattern from technician (one at a time).

Variation: Patient strings series of beads copying total pattern from technician.

Coloring

Scribbling on paper with pencil.

Variation: With crayons.

Variation: With finger paints.

Walks on Grounds

This differs from the primary activity in that objects of interest are brought to attention of children.

Example: Grass, trees, birds, people, cars, trucks, fire hydrants, weather, sky, etc.

ADVANCED ACTIVITIES

Marching

Variation: Stamp feet as they march.

Variation: Clap hands as they march.

Variation: Dwarfs—march in squatting position, making self as small as possible.

Variation: Giants—march on tiptoes, hold hands high in air, reaching up as high as possible.

Variation: Dolls—march stiff legged and with bodies rigid like dolls.

Variation: Rooster—walk like a rooster with knee lifted high and leg stretched forward.

Variation: Kangaroo—walk like a kangaroo, elbows close to body, forearm up, chest high, and hands drooping. In this position move with short jumps.

Variation: Major—strut with high knee action like a drum major.

Coloring—Coloring on a given area of paper with crayons. Example: Filling in circle, square made by Technician on paper before distributing.

Storytelling—Technician reads simple story to group of children.
Length of story—about 5 minute story—should be about experiences of children and family life. Story told should be well illustrated and references to picture should be made by Technician. Technician may also make up interesting stories to fit children's need; an action story or quiet story.

Cutting—Learning to handle scissors, not following any lines or pattern.
This takes time.

Variation: Following a broad, straight line on paper.

Variation: Following a broad, curved line on paper.

Variation: Cutting out simple objects—previously colored, an apple, ball, etc.

Variation: Pictures and figures from magazines, catalogues, and greeting cards.

Pasting

Using one finger to spread paste, a little at a time.

Using wide paste brush.

Making paper chain from paper strips pasted together.

Making designs from colored squares and circles.

Making interesting scrapbooks.

Action Songs

The Farmer in the Dell
The Farmer in the Dell
The Farmer in the Dell
Hi Ho the Dairy-O
The Farmer in the Dell
The Farmer Takes a wife
The Wife takes a child
The child takes a nurse
The nurse takes a dog
The dog takes a cat
The cat takes the rat
The rat takes the cheese
The cheese stands alone

Children form a circle holding hands, facing in, singing or chanting the songs as the circle revolves around a person in the center of the circle (the farmer). As the chant or singing progresses the person in the center (the farmer) chooses someone from the circle to be the wife. This person (wife) disengages from the circle and joins farmer in the center as the circle continues to revolve and go on to next verse. Wife then chooses child from circle, etc.

Variation: Add pantomime—each character acts out his part in center circle . . .

The Farmer: milks a cow
The Wife: feeds chickens
The Child: cries
The Nurse: helps child
The Dog: is on hands, knees and barks
The Cat: paws at dog
The Rat: runs from cat
The Cheese: stands still

Have all children help each time to try to imagine new situations.

Pop Goes the Weasel
All around the cobblers' bench
The monkey chased the weasel

The monkey though 'twas all in fun
    Pop! goes the weasel
Children join hands in circle, singing, circling, and on "Pop"
drop hands and clap.

Looby Loo

1. I put my right hand in
   I take my right hand out
   I give my hand a shake, shake, shake
   And turn myself about
   Chorus:
   Here we go Looby Loo
   Here we go Looby light
   Here we go Looby Loo
   All on a Saturday night

2. I put my left hand in
   I take my left hand out
   I give my hand a shake, shake, shake
   And turn myself about
   Repeat chorus

3. I put my right foot in
   I take my right foot out
   I give my foot a shake,
      shake, shake
   And turn myself about.
   Repeat chorus

4. I put my left foot in
   I take my left foot out
   I give my foot a shake, shake, shake
   And turn myself about
   Repeat chorus

5. I put my whole self in
   I take my whole self out
   I give myself a shake,
      shake, shake
   And turn myself about
   Repeat chorus

Children form circle, holding hands, facing in, singing or chanting
the song, as the circle revolves. When the chorus is finished, they

stop, drop hands, and imitate motions given in verse. (Example: Right hand is extended into circle, is brought out of the circle behind child, is brought back in front and shaken three times and child turns himself around in place and grabs hands and goes into chorus again).

Mulberry Bush

Here we go round the mulberry bush, the mulberry bush, the mulberry bush

Here we go round the mulberry bush so early in the morning.

Variations:

1. This is the way we wash our face.
   (scrubbing motion on face)
   (Chorus)
2. This is the way we wash our hands.
   (actions likewise)
   (Chorus)
3. This is the way we brush our teeth.
   (Chorus)
4. This is the way we comb our hair.
   (Chorus)
5. This is the way we tie our shoes.
   (Chorus)
6. This is the way we wash our clothes.
   (Chorus)
7. This is the way we iron our clothes.
   (Chorus)

Variations unlimited . . .

ACTION GAMES

Tag

Tag is where one person is "It" and this individual tries to tag other players thus making the tagged play "It."

Variations: *Squat Tag*—Players may not be tagged as long as they are in a squat position.

Variation: *Poison Tag*—Player tagged must hold place where he was tagged with his left (or right) hand.

Variation: *Line Tag*—As the 1st player is tagged, he joins hands with "It" and either end of the line may tag. As 2nd, 3rd, etc. players are tagged, only the two end players may tag . . . ("It is always on one end and the newest tagged.)

Mouse Trap

Played like London Bridge. Two players join hands to form an arch— The "Mouse Trap." Others playing are "mice" who skip or run in single line under the arch "Mouse Trap." When the Leader calls "Snap!" the "Mouse Trap" falls and catches the mouse going under. The "mouse" that is caught stands aside until another "mouse" is caught and then they form another trap. Game continues with new traps being formed until one "mouse" is left!

Appendix B

WHAT MENTAL AGE OF 5 CAN DO

Boys

1. Wash dishes
2. Sandpaper furniture
3. Scrub and polish floors
4. Food and fold from mangle
5. Simple domestic work
6. Brushmaker's assistant
7. Handle cinders and garbage
8. Make nets
9. Cut rags in accurate strips

Girls

1. Follow a pattern in simple sewing
2. Pare vegetables
3. Cut rags in accurate strips
4. Wash dishes by hand
5. Sew rag carpet

WHAT MENTAL AGE OF 6 CAN DO

Boys

1. Mow lawn
2. Kitchen scullery
3. Mix cement
4. Handle freight
5. Brush making
6. Simple laundry work
7. Assist brick mason

Girls

1. Crochet open mesh
2. Weave rag rug with pattern
3. Simple laundry work
4. Operate mangle
5. Fold clothing

Courtesy Rehabilitation Services Series No. 123 booklet "Vocational Rehabilitation of the Mentally Retarded," U. S. Department of Health, Education and Welfare, Office of Vocational Rehabilitation, Washington, D. C. Salvatore G. DiMichael, Editor.

WHAT MENTAL AGE OF 7 CAN DO

Boys

1. Rough painting
2. Simple shoe repairing
3. Drive two-horse team
4. Plow
5. Blacksmith
6. Cane chair
7. Make brooms
8. Simple carpentry
9. Domestic work

Girls

1. Knit neckties and scarves
2. Plain and Italian hemstitching
3. Cross stitch
4. Braid
5. Sew rags for rugs
6. Simple domestic work
7. Hand ironing
8. Simple packing of small articles

WHAT MENTAL AGE OF 8 CAN DO

Boys

1. Handle coal, ashes
2. Pitch and load hay
3. General farm work
4. PAINT OUTSIDE and interior
5. Cut hair and shave
6. Shingle and set glass
7. Make wooden toys
8. Make nets
9. Garden work
10. Repair mattresses

Girls

1. Stitch neckties
2. Make baskets
3. Operate bead loom
4. Stencil work
5. Dress doll without help
6. Operate scarf loom
7. Make dresses cut out by others
8. Plain ironing
9. High grade domestic work
10. Hand weaving and knitting

WHAT MENTAL AGE OF 9 CAN DO

Boys

1. Entire process of broom making
2. Foot power printing press
3. Block paper into pads
4. Repair furniture
5. Paint toys
6. Higher processes of shoe repairing
7. Harvest vegetables and fruit
8. Mattress and pillow making
9. Learn an alto horn and manipulate drums
10. Fancy brushmaking

Girls

1. Knit stockings and mittens
2. Fancy basket making
3. Cloth toy making
4. Pottery making
5. Operate automatic rug loom
6. Cut out and make dresses
7. Plain cooking
8. Pillow lace making
9. Sew mounts on cardboard
10. Sew buttons
11. Make novelties
12. Sew lining (hat industry)

WHAT MENTAL AGE OF 10 CAN DO

Boys

1. Setting and sorting type
2. Sign painting
3. Electrician assistant
4. Steam fitters assistant
5. Form making for cement and floors
6. Shellacking and varnishing
7. Learn bass horn and cornet
8. Laundry work (detailed)
9. Garden work (detailed)
10. Farm work and dairying

Girls

1. Raffia and reed work pattern
2. Basketry
3. Swedish embroidery
4. Operate sweater machine
5. Operate looper for stocking toes
6. Starching and polishing (laundry)
7. Fancy laundry work
8. Fancy cooking (candy and cookies)
9. Canning
10. Learn cornet and saxophone

WHAT MENTAL AGES OF 11 AND 12 CAN DO

Boys	*Girls*
1. Competent janitors	1. Sew garters and powder puffs
2. Stockkeeping	2. Sew wire edges and facing in hats
3. Keep small store	3. Simple library work
4. Labeling and checking	4. Italian cut work embroidery
5. Greenhouse attendant	5. Power sealing in canning plant
6. Lawn caretaker	6. Learn first violin, cello, flute, and clarinet

DISORDERS OF PSYCHOGENIC ORIGIN OR WITHOUT CLEARLY DEFINED PHYSICAL CAUSE OR STRUCTURAL CHANGE IN THE BRAIN*

I. *Involutional Psychotic Reaction*

Depressions occurring in the involutional period, usually in persons who are compulsive. Typical symptoms are worry, intractable insomnia, guilt, anxiety, agitation, delusional ideas, somatic preoccupation that may become delusional. Depression or paranoid ideas may dominate the reaction pattern.

II. *Affective Reactions*

A. Manic depressive reactions.

Characterized by mood swings, with a tendency to remission and recurrence and may be accompanied by secondary symptoms of illusions, delusions, and hallucinations.

1. Manic depressive reaction, manic type.

Characterized by elation or irritability, circumstantially, flight of ideas, overactivity. Momentary or transient depression may occur.

2. Manic depressive reaction, depressed type.

Characterized by mood depression, mental and motor retardation, uneasiness and apprehension. Perplexity, stupor, or agitation may occur.

3. Manic depressive reaction, other.

Reactions showing mixture of two preceding, or continuous alteration of the two. Other variants, such as manic stupor or unproductive mania, are included.

---

*Quoted from the American Psychiatric Association's Manual, *Diagnostic and Statistical Manual for Mental Disorders.*

III. *Schizophrenic Reactions*
  A. Schizophrenic reaction, simple type.
     Characterized by reduction in external attachments and by impoverishment of human relationships. Apathy and indifference occur. Severity of symptoms increase over a long period of time with mental deterioration. Hallucinations and delusions are infrequent.
  B. Schizophrenic reaction, hebephrenic type.
     Typical symptoms are inappropriate and shallow affect, silly behavior and mannerisms, giggling, delusions, hallucinations, and regressive behavior.
  C. Schizophrenic reaction, catatonic type.
     Motor behavior is significant in this group. Generalized inhibition is shown in stupor, mutism, negativism, and waxy flexibility. Excessive motor activity and excitement also occur.
  D. Schizophrenic reaction, paranoid type.
     The paranoid schizophrenic reaction is characterized by autistic, unrealistic thinking, delusions of persecution and/or delusions of grandeur, ideas of reference, and hallucinations. Behavior is unpredictable, but an underlying hostility and aggression are often constant.
  E. Schizophrenic reaction, acute undifferentiated type.
     An acute episode that tends to clear, including a wide variety or schizophrenic symptoms. These include confused thinking, emotional upheaval, perplexity, ideas of reference, fear and dream states, and dissociative phenomena.
  F. Schizophrenic reaction, chronic undifferentiated type.
     Characterized by chronicity and mixed symptomatology of the schizophrenic variety.
  G. Schizophrenic reaction, schizo-affective type.
     This category includes those who show significant admixtures of schizophrenic and affective reactions.
  H. Schizophrenic reaction, childhood type.
     Reactions occurring before puberty.
IV. *Paranoid Reactions*
   Characterized by persistent delusions, usually persecutory or grandiose; emotional response consistent with ideas held and by good intellectual preservation.

Appendix D

THE TECHNIQUE OF REMOTIVATION*

In its original form, Remotivation is based on five essential steps. In practice, it has been demonstrated that adherence to these five steps creates a more stable and lasting program. For the psychiatric aide, full knowledge and appreciation of these steps provides him with a "stepping-off" point, a level of continuity, and a hopeful and promising conclusion.

In utilizing the five steps, it is important that the psychiatric aide know why he has been selected to work with his patients in this individual and special way. In most mental illnesses there are parts of the patient's original personality which remain relatively untouched. In other words, in certain areas, his personality—and his interests—have remained healthy. Frequently, the "untouched parts" have to do with everyday, ordinary things which many of us take for granted—the way a tree grows, the history of our native state, what wares we might find in a department store, what smoke means in our daily lives, what makes weather, and the multitude of things with which we live and people with whom we must interact.

The aide should keep in mind however, that he is not "teaching" patients—although it is true that both patient and aide do learn from these sessions. These are not "classes." They are group meetings in which a sharing or pooling of ideas promotes personal interaction between aide and patients, and among patients themselves. Thus, although the aide does not have to "study" and cram his head full of "facts and figures," it helps to look up and review certain subjects

---

*Quoted from the manual *Remotivation Technique,* written by Alice M. Robinson, R.N., M.S. by permission of: American Psychiatric Association Mental Hospital Service and the Smith Kline and French Foundation Remotivation Project.

in order to provide a maximum background of interesting information on the selected topic.

Selection of the Group

The patient group should be selected by the ward physician, the ward, nurse, and the psychiatric aide. Approximately fifteen patients comprise an "ideal size group." Certain limits on Remotivation must be considered in selecting patients: (1) the type of ward (admitting or acute; continued treatment; senile and/or infirmary; and convalescent); (2) the designation and extent of the patients' various illnesses, and (3) the warmth and skillfulness of the remotivation aide. According to one of the aides actively engaged in this type of program: "It is usually wise to include one or two patients you know will talk and help you 'carry the ball' during the session." It is also advisable not to include patients who are engaged in a number of other activities, although no patient can legitimately be excluded.

The Five Steps

As previously stated, the "five steps" form the core of remotivation and, in a sense, make it a special technique. The psychiatric aide-leader should thoroughly familiarize himself with these five steps through lectures, demonstrations, and sufficient practice sessions under supervision. The title of each of the five steps gives a clue to the gist of its performance. Since remotivation group meetings usually last about 50 minutes to an hour, a suggested span will be included for each step.

The Climate of Acceptance (5 min.)

In this first step, the aide-leader (who is standing) addresses the group in general, and may initially express his appreciation to the group for coming to the session. He then moves slowly around the circle greeting each patient warmly and individually, by name. If there is a new patient in the group or the aide is unsure of the patient's name, he may introduce himself and ask the patient's name. He can comment on the weather, on a patient's dress or haircut, or any little appropriate comment which establishes a person-to-person contact with that particular patient. Introductory remarks should be pleasant and objective.

The purpose of this first step is the establishment of a comfortable, relaxed atmosphere for the patients and the aide. If the aide can think of himself as a fellow participant and an interested learner, he is psychologically better prepared to guide the subsequent group discussion. (In the light of the above suggestions for creating a climate of acceptance, it goes without saying that patients should not be forced to attend remotivation meetings. The aide can, however, encourage the patient to attend the succeding meetings and would do well to approach the resisting patient before the start of the next meeting.)

The first step has already accomplished something for the patient. He is experiencing something different, which takes him away from the usual routine and which involves him directly within a group of his fellows.

A Bridge to Reality (15 min.)

In the Remotivation technique as originally developed, the bridge to reality was created by the reading of objective poetry. Although this may, at first, seem rather a strange way to try to reach the mentally sick patient, it works surprisingly well in practice.

In one recently observed session, a robust "he-man" aide whose topic was baseball began to read the ever-famous, "Casey at the Bat." The patient group was comprised of young adult men from an acute admitting ward, and they listened intently to the first lines read by the aide-leader. When he began passing the poem around, asking each patient to read a few lines, they responded enthusiastically, and even inquired as to the name of the poet. In another session, conducted for about 15 working men patients, the aide-leader and the patients read Carl Sandburg's "Smoke and Steel," which immediately set the group off on a lively discussion about working in the steel mills. In still another session (this patient group consisting of severely regressed schizophrenic women), the aide began to read Joyce Kilmer's "Trees" and thereby set the stage for a verbal examination of birds—particularly the first Spring robins and the perennial pigeons observed by the patients as they apparently sat listless in the yard on nice days.

If poetry is used in the second step, it should be simple, rhythmic, and appropriate to the selected topic. (Although, as suggested, the paper-bound Anthology of Verse contained many usable poems, the aide would do well to start his own collection of poems, "keeping an eye open" for poems in everyday magazines—frequently seasonal and frequently related to current events. In one observed session, a patient asked whether or not anyone had written a poem about "sputnik.")

Rather than poetry, the aide-leader may wish to start a session with a famous quotation or with a newspaper item (i.e., women's fashion trends, a new birth at the zoo, or the progress of a national golf tournament).

It is important during this second step, and, in fact, throughout the session for the aid-leader to move around he group as he reads, and to encourage individual patients to read parts of the selected poem or article.

Sharing the World We Live In (15 min.)

The purpose of this third step is the development of the topic covered by the group. This is accomplished by means of objective questions which are carefully planned. (In several groups observed, the aide-leaders had written down ten or twelve questions, and unselfconsciously referred to these questions as the discussion progressed. Such preplanned questions serve to keep the group "on the track" and eliminate the tendency to "go with the group" thereby getting away from the topic.)

One of the most effective methods of fostering patient interest in the subject at hand is the use of related "props." These can consist of pictures cut out of magazines, maps, historical pamphlets, plants, samples of dress materials—the possibilities are endless. (One aide-leader brought in her Mexican Chihauhua to the delight of her patient group!) To quote again, from an aide-leader's notes: "There are almost no limitations on the selection of subject matter, as long as it remains objective and is one in which it can be reasonably certain there will be patient interest, and about which they have some knowledge and . . . will be able to some extent to answer questions."

Some of the more obvious limitations on the selection of subject matter would include such topics as religion, sex, prejudice, marital problems, family relationships and similar "touchy" areas.

An Appreciation of the Work of the World (15 min.)

This fourth step in most instances, is designed to prompt the patient into thinking about work in relation to himself. The skillful aide-leader manipulates the conclusion of the third step (at the proper time) into a discussion of the value of work, and any jobs which are related to the planned topic. (In senile or infirm groups, and in groups of severely regressed and deteriorated patients, this step may quite reasonably be omitted. However, in one observed group composed of elderly "chair-bound" men, the aide-leader was able to initiate rather lively discussion of jobs which had been held by these patients in the past!)

As in the above example, some of the patients may be able to give the group interesting information as to how a certain commodity is produced or how a specific job is done. In other instances, the aide-leader may ask what job a patient might prefer if given a choice in a particular work situation. (In a group of "disturbed" women patients in an active treatment ward, the aide-leader had been showing magazine cutouts of various products which are usually found in a large department store. After circulating the pictures she asked each individual patient in which department of the store she might like to work—provided she was given a choice. Although one or two patients facetiously named the "candy department" or the "complaint department," most of the answers provided valuable clues as to the patient's real work interest. At a future date, it would be helpful for the aide-leader to pass on such information to the ward physician and/or the industrial therapist.)

The Climate of Appreciation (5 min.)

Finally, this fifth and last step enables the aide-leader to express his enjoyment of the group and his pleasure that the patients were able to come to the session. This is the time for him to indicate plans for the next session, thus providing the patients with a sense of continuity and with something to which they can look forward.

The Meeting Plan

In the process of studying the five steps, it becomes obvious that the aide-leader who draws up even a brief "meeting plan" will be better prepared to "remotivate" patients throughout each session.

Appendix E

SYLLABUS ON MENTAL RETARDATION*

DIAGNOSTIC CLASSIFICATIONS

I. *Cerebral Lipoidosis, Infantile (Tay-Sachs' Disease)*

A. This is a condition known by many names. The old name is amaurotic familial idiocy. There are several forms of this condition occurring at different age groups. *Amaurosis* means blindness, familial means that it occurs in families and idiocy refers to a severe degree of mental retardation. The condition is progressive. The child seems to be normal at birth and during the first six months of life. The initial symptoms generally do not occur before the age of 6 months and then the child progressively deteriorates until death.

II. *Galactosemia*

A. Characterized by congenital disorder of metabolism of carbohydrates which results in an accumulation of galactose (a form of sugar) in the blood stream.

B. Baby in good condition at birth but on a milk diet soon begins to show symptoms.

C. Jaundice and vomiting are common and in spite of an insatiable appetite the child shows evidence of malnutrition.

---

*Manual on Terminology and Classification in Mental Retardation prepared by the American Association on Mental Deficiency.

III. Gargoylism (Hurler's Disease)

A. Some signs may be evident at birth; there is head enlargement and limitation of joint movements.

B. The gargoyl has a large head with a protruding forehead which is far out of proportion with the stunted body, the eyebrows are bushy and the nose saddle shaped. The features are coarse and heavy with a deep crease between lower lip and chin. Degree of retardation ranges from minimal to severe, usually being evident by time child is two years of age.

IV. Hydrocephalous

A. Refers to the condition in which the head becomes unusually large due to the over-production and collection of spinal fluid within the brain.

V. Hypertelorism (Greig's Disease)

A. Distance between eyes is increased, in extreme cases so much so that the eyes appear to be on the sides of the face rather than in the normal frontal position. Hare lip and cleft palate are frequently present.

VI. Hypothyroidism

A. May be divided into congenital (born with) and acquired types as a cause of retardation.

B. Due to lack of thyroid secretion.

VII. Kernicterus, Associated with Retardation

A. May follow severe jaundice in the newborn.

B. Frequently due to Rh incompatability.

VIII. Mental Retardation Associated with Emotional Disturbances

A. This applies to cases of retardation associated with a history of a prolonged period of emotional disturbance dating from an early age.

B. It is believed that the emotional disturbance must be extremely severe in order to have any causal relationship to mental retardation.

IX. Mental Retardation Associated with Environmental Deprivation

A. In some instances borderline or mild degrees of mental retardation may be attributed to a deprivation at an early age of opportunity for learning experiences which are essential for adequate functioning in our culture.

X. Mental Retardation as a result of the mother having an infection before child is born; three of which are:

A. Rubella (German Measles)
   1. May result if mother contracts rubella during first 3 months of pregnancy.
   2. May result in a variety of congenital defects such as deafness, cataracts, heart defects or mental defect.
B. Syphilis
   1. If a mother has syphilis which has been untreated she may pass it on to her unborn baby.
C. Toxoplasmosis
   1. The unborn child contracts this disease if the mother has an infection caused by the organism *Toxoplasma*.

XI. Mental Retardation Resulting from Infection

A. Various infecting agents that involve the brain or its covering, called the meninges, may lead to mental retardation.
   1. Virus encephalitis is one of the most common types, occurring when the human is an infant or child. The individual may recover from the acute stages of the disease only to develop the complications of mental retardation.

XII. Microcephaly

A. This term is reserved for cases with an adult head circumference of 17 inches or less. Correspondingly for chil-

dren, it is 13 inches at 6 months, 14 inches at 1 year
and 15 inches at 2 years.
B. Contrast between the small cranium and the relatively
well-developed face is diagnostic.
C. Moderate to severe retardation is present.

XIII. *Mongolism (Down's Syndrome)*

A. Most common of so-called clinical types of mental retardation.
B. Latest research reports indicate that one of the determi-
nant factors causing this condition is an extra chromosome,
there being 47 instead of the normal 46.
C. Tongue tends to protrude from mouth, skin lacks normal
elasticity, hands and feet are broad and clumsy and the
little finger tends to be very short and curve inward.
There are characteristic palm and finger prints. In approximately 10 per cent of cases there is congenital heart
defect.
D. Degree of retardation ranges from moderate to severe.

XIV. *Neurofibromatosis (von Recklinghausen's Disease)*

A. Characterized by pigmentation of the skin and tumors of
the nerve trunk and skin. "Cafe au lait" patches which
vary greatly in size and in the area of the trunk covered
are present in almost all cases. Epilepsy may also be
present.

XV. *Oxycephaly*

A. Characterized by a tower or steeple-shaped skull consisting of a high narrow forehead which slopes to a point.
B. Vision, hearing and smell may be impaired.

XVI. *Prenatal Injury*

A. Difficulties during labor increase the probability of damage to the infant's brain at birth.
B. Use of xrays on the mother during the first three months
of pregnancy may result in retardation of varying degrees
of severity.

INDEX

problem drinker, 202
psychotherapy, 107, 166, 170
religious training, 103
remotivation, 236. *Also see*
  Appendix D
restraints, seclusion, 84
seizures, patients, 40, 42, 43
self-feeding, 55
shampooing, shaving, 78
shock therapies, 193
spastic patient, the, 40
suicide, prevention of, 195-197
toothbrushing, 73
vocational training, 98, 99, 102, 105
volunteers, 106
ward, the, 45
Psychiatrist, 121
Psychiatry, definition of, 121
Psychologist, 7, 32, 121, 204
Psychology, 121
Psychoneuroses, the, 153
  anxiety states, 154, 155
  conversion reaction, 156
  depressive reaction, 155, 156
  obsessive-compulsive reaction, 155
  phobic reaction, 155
Psychopath, sexual, 206
Psychoses, the, 156
  functional, 156, 157
  involutional depression, 157
  manic-depressive, 157
  paranoid, 158
  schizophrenia, 158, 159, 160
  organic, 156, 157
Psychosomatic, definition of, 123
Psychosurgery, 164, 165
Psychotherapy, 107, 131
Pulse, 62, 63

Q

Quotient, intelligence, 31, 32
  social, 32

R

Rapport, 123
Rationalization, 149
Reaction, conversion, 156
  depressive, 155, 156
  obsessive-compulsive, 155

phobic, 155
Reading, selected, 211-214
Reality, contact with, 188-189
Records, 118
Regularity, in habit training, 51
Regurgitation, 57
Rehabilitation therapists, 8
Religious training, 103, 105
Remission, 123
Remotivation, technique of, 236. *Also
  see* Appendix D
Respiration, 62, 63
Repression, 146
Restraints, use of, 84, 89
Retarded, borderline, 30, 33
  mildly, 30, 33
  moderately, 33
  profoundly (gross), 34
  severely, 33
Room, day, 46
  dining, 47
Rumination, 58
Rush, Benjamin, 129, 201, 202

S

Scabies, 81
Schedule, example, 52
Schizophrenia, 158-160
  childhood, 183, 184
School, teacher, 7, 32
Seclusion, use of, 85
Seizures, 40, 124, 125. *Also see*
  Epilepsy
Sequin, Edward, 23, 25
Shock, insulin, 163
Shock, signs of, 90
Skills, motor, 10, 15
Skin, care of, 63, 65, 69
Social, criteria, 33
  growth, 27
  quotient, 32
  service workers, 6
  therapy, 166
Socialization, need for, 29
Sociopathic personality, 205
Somatic therapies, 162-165
Spastic, the, 38, 40
Stability, emotional, 30
Sterilization, 25, 26, 31